Intermittent Fasting: Your Ideal 7-day Intermittent Fasting Diet Plan to Lose Weight Now

By Susanne Bernard

Copyright 2018 - All Rights Reserved – Susanne Bernard
ALL RIGHTS RESERVED. No part of this publication may be reproduced or transmitted in any form whatsoever, electronic, or mechanical, including photocopying, recording, or by any informational storage or retrieval system without express written, dated and signed permission from the author.

Introduction:

I want to thank you and congratulate you for downloading the book, "Intermittent Fasting to Look and Feel Better".

Intermittent fasting or IF is a kind of eating technique that brings about a lot of health benefits to a person's overall health. Apart from the advantage of weight loss, this also paves the way to a healthier and stronger version of yourself.

This book contains proven steps and strategies on how to effectively use Intermittent Fasting in losing weight. If you've tried a lot of diet fads before and find it hard to maintain one, you probably have wondered what's the best diet to follow. The sheer number of different diets out there can be overwhelming and at times confusing. This is why Intermittent Fasting is becoming one of the go-to diets nowadays. For those who want to avoid passing fads that will work for a few days and then backfire and get you to an even worse shape than you were before, this book is for you.

Intermittent Fasting has been practiced for thousands of years. Did you know that you are also practicing this every day while you sleep through the night? There are many reasons why intermittent fasting is a great diet to adopt. It has numerous health benefits that include strengthening of the immune system, increasing longevity, calming of the mind, and helping you get to your ideal weight.

You may get the idea that fasting is going completely without food for several hours. There are specific fasting plans that you can follow. So if you wanted to learn more, go through the pages and start learning more about Intermittent Fasting.

Chapter 1: All about Intermittent fasting

Intermittent Fasting or IF encourages abstinence from food for a set period of time. This is also known as the non-feeding state that may last for up to 16 hours per cycle. This is followed by a brief period of eating and drinking specific food that will help in fat loss. This window is also referred to as the feeding state, thereby filling the gaps between cycles.

If the idea of not eating anything for 16 hours scares you, consider the fasting hours as your resting state as fasting usually begins when you retire for the night. In truth, Intermittent Fasting can be easily implemented if you practice eating an early dinner, and then have brunch the next day.

This long period of daily fasting helps the body to effectively burn off calories consumed during the feeding state. The most important benefit of all when you go fasting is that the stubborn fats are also burned off and are successfully converted into energy.

In order to make sure that weight loss is achieved, it is important that you create your own fasting schedule that you can religiously adhere to and apply in your current lifestyle. The time you're fasting (whether night or day) doesn't really matter. What matters is that you know for yourself that you can maintain the schedule until you've reached your personal goal.

Shifting from one fasting to another will put a toll on your digestive system. This will also increase the chances of binge eating during your unguarded moments, which will only lead to further weight gain.

Also, this may pose minor acid reflux, peptic ulcers, dyspepsia, and the like. This is why it is vital that you follow your Intermittent Fasting schedule accurately. And because the body's system isn't into using most of its energy into digestion during the resting period, rejuvenation and healing happen in the cellular level.

If this continues, this will help strengthen your immune system and overall health. This can also pave the way for developing lean muscles for a leaner physique.

If you're a beginner, you may start with a month's worth of trial. Before you fast, prepare your body by abstaining from food within 8 hours. Normally, Intermittent Fasting is a 16-hour fast. But for the first few days, you may start with an 8-12 hours fast.

Once you have successfully pulled through your trial IF, you can gradually lengthen your non-feeding state. From 8 hours, you may prolong it to 10, 12, 14, and 16.

What You Should Eat

The best thing about Intermittent Fasting is that there are no food restrictions. You can still eat the food that you like provided that you do it in moderation and consume them within your feedings state.

Intermittent Fasting does not also require calorie counting. However, you still have to watch what you eat if you want to lose weight fast.

Your Go-to Food List

✓ Fresh fruits and vegetables – vegetables are low in calories and can fill you up easily. As for fruits, eat only smaller portions of fruits that are high in sugar and fat such as banana and avocado.

✓ Proteins – if you're into muscle building, you should consume a higher amount of protein-rich food such as beans and legumes, beef, lean pork, chicken, eggs, dairy, seafood, nuts, and seeds.

✓ Mushrooms – these are low in fat and can be a good addition to your meals.

Food to Avoid

- Fast food – almost everything sold in fastfood should be avoided when you are in intermittent fasting. This is because these food are oily, salty, and starchy. Regular consumption can cause heart disease because fast food chains usually use hydrogenated oils.
- Processed food – this generally consists of sausages, hotdogs, chicken nuggets, and luncheon meat among others. These food no longer contain vital nutrients from the original meat

and are often made from poor quality meat. Apart from this, processed food also contains too much salt and food additives.
- Pre-packed food – these are frozen and microwaveable meals that contain high levels of preservatives, sweeteners, and sodium that only promote weight gain.
- Commercially-baked bread and pastries – these baked goodies contain refined starches and simple carbs that are absorbed in the stomach lining and become blood sugar. This sudden stream of sugar in the bloodstream makes the pancreas release insulin. Unfortunately, when a person overindulges in sweets, blood sugar remains high throughout the day. Insulin hormones are either overwhelmed by the surge and fail to function or the body stops producing insulin completely. When that happens, the brain will not receive its share of glucose, which is its source of sustenance.

Chapter 2 – Benefits of Intermittent Fasting

The main benefit of Intermittent Fasting is that you get to lose weight naturally. But when done correctly, IF can also help you:

Reduce the effects of Type II diabetes

According to the World Health Organization, about 380 million people are suffering from the complications of diabetes. Type II diabetes begins with insulin resistance. It is due mainly of excessive consumption of simple carbohydrates. This often manifests in people who are obese and with a sedentary lifestyles. Insulin resistance happens when the bloodstream is oversaturated with simple carbs. Simple carbs are usually found in processed food, sodas, cakes, sweets, and fast food. These are also present in refined grains such as white rice, white pasta, instant oats, and white flour among others.

When a person consumes high amounts of simple carbs, insulin in the bloodstream is supposed to absorb and convert these into useable calories. But this does not happen all the time. Insulin cells become overwhelmed with blood sugar. People with high blood sugar are always hungry especially after a heavy meal. Some even experience unusual food cravings during odd hours.

During the fasting state, the level of insulin stabilizes. And since there is lack of calorie intake, the body utilizes whatever sugar is left in the bloodstream. These are quickly converted into usable energy. This state will help to lower down blood sugar levels, and makes it easier to process excess calories out of the system.

Reduce the risk of cancer

According to studies, fasting for 8 to 16 hours lowers the risk of cancer of the adipose tissues, cancer of the epithelial cells/lining such as in prostate, colon, and bladder. Lowers the risk of leukemia, cancer of the lymph nodes, cancer of the connective tissues, and germ cell tumor that usually grows in male and female reproductive organs.

Intermittent fasting helps in lowering the risk of cancer cells to other healthy organs. This is made possible because there is effective cleansing of the blood and eliminating toxins out of the body.

Increase muscle mass

Overeating and overindulging makes it difficult for the body to process excess food. Given this, it has no other choice but to continue making adipose tissues for all unwanted calories. Intermittent fasting helps the body gradually burn off calories in the adipose tissues. These are the stubborn fats that are difficult to lose even if you exercise. During fasting, the body starts working with its other energy sources. Over time, the body uses stored calories in the adipose tissues. This process helps the body develop leaner muscle mass.

Apart from this, a good amount of sleep and intermittent fasting combination will give you a lot of energy the next day. You can use that energy for exercise, which will help in developing leaner muscle mass.

Fasting is easier to follow

Some diets fads out there are quite difficult to follow. Some are very restrictive such as counting calories, drinking only juices, listing down corresponding amount of food, and eliminating major food groups from your daily meals such as carbohydrates or proteins.

You need not do all these when you do intermittent fasting. You can keep eating your favorite food as long as you give your body enough time to process them.

Of course, we recommend healthy food options especially if you want to lose weight quickly.

Chapter 3 – different Methods of Intermittent fasting

Intermittent fasting can be done in more ways than one. The method that you are going to follow will only depend on what you think is right for you. Learn more about the different methods and know which one is for you.

1. 16/8 Method

This is also known as the Leangains method, which makes you fast for 14-16 hours every day and eat only during the remaining 8 to 10 hours. You may skip breakfast and only eat between 12 noon to 8 pm.

During the fasting period (from night to morning), any calorie-laden food are not allowed. It would be best if you would just drink water or black coffee with calorie-free sweeteners. If you would like to stick to this timeframe, remember to stick with it so your hormones may be able to function properly.

Always be mindful of what you eat even if you're on intermittent fasting. Pro tip: eat carbohydrates if you're going to exercise or perfume some physical activity. Eat fat on days when you don't feel like exercising. Apart from this, majority of the food that you have to eat should be consists of whole, unprocessed ones.

2. Alternate Day Fasting

This requires fasting on alternate days of the week. For example, you can eat breakfast on Monday and then fast for the next 24 hours. You will have your next meal on Tuesday morning. Before Wednesday breakfast time, you can eat the entire time and fast again for another 24 hours after your last meal on Wednesday breakfast. You then go on a longer periods of fasting while eating at least one meal each day of the week.

This is said to be more beneficial to the body you are on an eating break for a longer period of time. This will also make it easier for you to lose weight since there is less calories consumed enabling you to lose those fats quickly.

5. The 5:2 Diet

This method of fasting is similar to the Alternate Day Intermittent Fasting. The only difference is that you are allowed to eat small portions during your fasting periods. For 2 days in a week, you are only allowed to consume 500 to 600 calories. The rest of the week for five days, you can eat your usual meals. The method is to consume small amounts of food one day and eat normally on the next day.

To make the down days manageable, try having replacement shakes that can be sipped the entire day. These shakes are fortified with essential nutrients. But you are only allowed to have replacement shakes during the first two weeks of this approach to intermittent fasting. During the down days, eat real food and eat normally during your up days.

This method of Intermittent Fasting is recommended for those who want to lose weight. According to research, cutting down your calories by at least 20 percent results in 2 and half pounds of weight loss each week.

Eat-Stop-Eat Intermittent Fasting

This means that you have to fast for 24 hours once or twice a week. You can do this by not eating at dinner one day until the next dinnertime the following day. This 24 hour fast requires you not to eat any food except from water and other calorie-free beverages.

The reason for this schedule is that it reduces your overall calorie intake. There are no restrictions to what you can eat, but only to how often. If you want to lose weight more quickly or improve your body composition, you should integrate regular exercises, particularly resistance training. If you find it hard to not eat for 24 hours straight, you need not be hard on yourself since IF is a flexible program.

You may gradually increase your fasting period from 14 hours to 16, 18, 20 and 24 gradually. It is easier to start fasting during your busy time.

The Warrior Diet

This method requires you to not eat for 20 hours each day and only eat one large meal every night. This synchronizes with circadian rhythms as we are naturally designed for night eating. This is also about "undereating", which is meant to promote alertness, boost energy, and facilitate fat-burning.

The 4-hour feeding window, known as the "overeating" phase is done at night to help the body to recuperate. This promotes digestion, relaxation, and calmness. The nutrients from the large meal that you have consumed helps in the body's growth and repair.

Also, it is imperative that you follow the order of eating specific food groups. Start your meals with vegetables, then proteins, and then finally fats.

Chapter 4 – Diet Plan

Diet Plan: How Many Meals per Day

The number of meals that you are allowed to consume is subjective. If you are a beginner, it might be easier to eat three full meals for now. You can tweak this later on when your body has already adjusted to your fasting schedule. Some who are already experienced in fasting eat two full meals a day, while others would stretch two to three snacks during their feeding state, with one full meal in between.

Apart from this, you also need to lessen your calorie intake if you want to lose weight. But if you're trying to bulk up on muscles, you need a few more calories.

Just remember that there should be no solid food during the non-feeding phase. Of course, water is an exception. If you plan on working out during your fasting period, you may consume small amounts of coffee or milk.

It is recommended that you consume your heaviest meal after exercising. Your body will start craving for sustenance soon after.

Other things you need to take note of:

- Dark, whole grain bread is processed by the body at a slower rate and is considered rich in fiber.
- If you want to eat carbohydrates, choose the dark-colored whole grains over white flour. This is because white flour is usually processed by the body as simple sugars.
- Consuming small amounts of whole grain helps stabilize blood sugar level. Regular consumption promotes better bowel movement, too.
- Make sure to keep an eye on beverages that you consume during your feeding state. Everything else that contains calories may slow down your weight loss.
- Every once in a while, it's fine to eat some bacon. Just don't go

overboard.

The Importance of Cheat Code

Using one will help simplify your daily meal preparations. For meat, 100 grams per meal will suffice. For fish fillets, 20 grams of protein will do.

140 grams or ¾ cup of cooked grains such as rice, pasta, noodles, or oats is equivalent to 100 grams of carbohydrates.

For vegetables, consume as much leafy greens as you want as these are mostly 70% water and contain very few calories in them. The best ones are cabbages, arugula, radicchio, beet tops, bok choi, spinach, dandelion greens, Swiss chard, endives, lettuce, kale, and napa cabbages among others. When cooking veggies, it is advised that you lightly prepare them like steaming, boiling, or grilling.

Finally, if you're going for salads with dressings, opt for the calorie-free dressings such as vinegar or lime and lemon juice.

Here's a Sample Meal Plan

Meal Plan for Days 1-7

Day 1
    Breakfast - Plantain with Soft Boiled Egg
    Lunch - Mixed Salad Greens
    Dinner - No-Bread Beef Bacon Burger
    Dessert/Snacks - Blueberry Scones

Day 2
    Breakfast - Wheat Cereal with Walnuts and Flaxseed
    Lunch - Asparagus and Green Peas Salad
    Dinner - Grilled Tempeh with Pineapple
    Dessert/Snacks - Vegan Ice Cream, Vanilla Flavor

Day 3
Breakfast - Scrambled Tofu
Lunch - Beef Chili and Beans
Dinner - Mushrooms, Chicken, and Chestnuts in Lettuce Wraps
Dessert/Snacks - Pecan Cilantro Pancakes
Day 4
Breakfast - Baby Bellas and Chicken Frittata
Lunch - Pumpkin and Apples Soup
Dinner - Fish Tofu and Shrimps Stir-Fry
Dessert/Snacks - Cashew Cheese
Day 5
Breakfast - Whole Wheat Sandwich with Spinach and Tomato
Lunch - Tuna Fillets with All Tomatoes Salad
Dinner - All Mushrooms Bake
Dessert/Snacks - Sausage and Beans Tacos
Day 6
Breakfast - Broccoli and Spinach Soup
Lunch - Cauliflower, Carrots, and Peas Curry
Dinner - Zucchini Roll-ups
Dessert/Snacks - Rosemary Flat Bread

Day 7
Breakfast - Spinach Pancakes
Lunch - Chicken Fillet Soup
Dinner - Artichoke, Beef and Bell Peppers Pie
Dessert/Snacks - Minty Cranberry Iced Tea

Chapter 5 – Mistakes

Subscribing to this diet takes a little getting used to. But if guidelines are followed to the letter, you sure will lose weight and fats along the way and the quickly and effectively.

Here are some common mistakes that most people do when they go on intermittent fasting:

- Never combine different diets with intermittent fasting as this can prove dangerous to your health. Follow one diet at a time. If you are going to switch to a new diet, give your body at least 2-3 weeks of rest and regain its equilibrium.
- During your feeding window, don't overeat on "healthy" food and drinks. This may sound a bit weird but think of it this way. There is a tendency to overindulge. Those who complain about not losing weight quickly enough is because there is a propensity to overindulge in "healthy" food items.

For example, a 100 grams dairy milk chocolate bar has 530 calories. You avoid that because it is unhealthy. So instead, you eat three 100 gram bars of granola. However, each bar has 391 calories. This means you have already consumed an estimate of 1,700 calories in just those 3 bars. The supposed to be healthy granola bar became unhealthier than the chocolate bar.

This is also the same with beverages. Did you know that a can of pineapple juice contains 440 calories? Let us suppose you consume four bottles in one day. So the next time you go for healthy eats, do not go overboard. Smaller portions are enough to make sure that you lose weight effectively during your fast.

- Say no to starvation. There is a big difference between fasting and starving. Fasting is abstaining from eating and drinking for a set amount of time. Starving is when your body feels deprived of life-sustaining food. When the body thinks that it is going through the first stages of malnutrition, it will spend its last energy reserve into creating more adipose tissues. Should the body survives this phase, it will just hoard all its newly obtained calories into the fat cells. And, what's worse is it will ensure that starvation will never happen again. This makes it even harder to lose adipose tissues around the midsection, thighs, shoulders, and butt.

- Don't eat processed food or beverages as part of your everyday meals. As much as possible, avoid canned fruits, packed fruit juices, bottled vegetables in brine, packed vegetables in water, and frozen fruits and vegetables.

- Don't settle for one goal alone. Instead, create a series of goals. For example, week 1, lose 1-2 pounds, weeks 3 -4, 3-5 pounds, and so on. Keep in mind, weight loss plateau is inevitable in almost all diets. It strikes weeks or months after successfully losing weight. This happens when your metabolism slows down and matches the number of calories you consume per day. This makes it difficult to lose weight afterwards. However, once you get over this phase, you can go back to your weight loss endeavor.

Chapter 6 – Recipes for Breakfast, salad, Lunch, Dinner, and Desserts/Snacks

Breakfast Recipes

Plantain with Soft Boiled Egg

Ingredients:

- 4 ripe plantains, quartered
- 2 eggs, soft-boiled
- ½ pound fresh kale, chopped
- Pinch sea salt
- Pinch of black pepper, to taste
- ½ tsp. olive oil

Directions:

1. Pour olive oil into a non-stick skillet.
2. Fry quartered plantains for 3 minutes or until golden brown. Turn down the heat to the lowest setting.
3. Stir in kale leaves. Stir well. Secure the lid and allow the kale leaves to cook for 2 minutes. Turn off the heat. Season with salt and pepper.
4. To serve, put desired amount of plantain hash into a plate. Serve with soft boiled egg and kale on the side.

Wheat Cereal with Walnuts and Flaxseed

Ingredients:

- 4 tablespoons wheat cereal
- 1 tablespoon ground flaxseed
- 1 tablespoon walnuts, chopped
- 1 tablespoon cranberries
- 1 cup evaporated milk, fat free
- ½ teaspoon vanilla extract

Directions:

1. Using a microwaveable-safe bowl, put together wheat cereal mad evaporated milk. Whisk well using a fork.
2. Place inside the microwave oven and heat for 2 minutes with 30 seconds interval.
3. Add in vanilla extract and flaxseed meal. Set aside.
4. Meanwhile, lightly grease a microwaveable-safe plate and spread the walnuts.
5. Place inside the microwave oven for 45 minutes on high pressure.
6. To serve, place an equal amount of cereal in a bowl. Put walnuts on top. Scatter cranberries.

Scrambled Tofu

Ingredients:

- 1 container soft tofu
- 2 tablespoons fresh basil, chopped
- 1/8 teaspoon turmeric
- 1 red onion, finely chopped
- 1 tablespoon fresh thyme, chopped
- 1 cup Cheddar cheese, reduced fat
- 2 tablespoons extra virgin olive oil
- Pinch of salt
- Pinch of pepper

Directions:

1. Heat the olive oil in a nonstick skillet. Saute onions for 3 minutes or until translucent. Crumble tofu into the pan. Season with turmeric, salt, and pepper. Cook for another 5 minutes whilst stirring frequently.
2. Remove pan from heat. Stir in basil, thyme, and cheese. Allow the cheese to melt before serving.

Baby Bellas and Chicken Frittata

Ingredients

- 8 baby bellas, minced
- 8 strips chicken breast, chopped
- 1 lb. parsnips
- 4 pieces of scallions, chopped
- Pinch of nutmeg
- 2 leeks, sliced
- 1 can of almond milk
- 1/4 teaspoon ground black pepper
- Olive oil

Directions

1. Cook the chicken strips in a non-stick pan; set aside.
2. Shred the parsnips; transfer to a mixing bowl.
3. Mix with the black pepper, nutmeg, kosher salt, leeks, and almond milk.
4. Transfer the parsnips mixture to a baking dish.
5. Top the parsnip mixture with crunchy duck strips, baby bellas and scallions.
6. Bake for one hour at 350 degrees F and serve when done.

Whole Wheat Sandwich with Spinach and Tomato

Ingredients:

- 4 whole wheat bread
- ¼ cup fresh spinach, cooked
- 1 tomato, sliced
- 1 hard-boiled egg, sliced
- 1 tablespoon mayonnaise, fat free
- Pinch of salt

Directions:

1. Set the whole wheat bread on a toaster over double sheet of foil. Top with spinach and tomato. Lay the egg slices and put a dollop of mayonnaise. Sprinkle seasoning.
2. Put sandwich under the broiler for 3 minutes until the mayonnaise turned light brown. Serve.

Broccoli and Spinach Soup

Ingredients:

- 1 head of broccoli, chopped
- 2 bunches spinach, chopped
- 7 oz silken tofu, drained
- 1 yellow onion, diced
- 1/2 tbsp. extra virgin olive oil
- 4 cups vegetable stock
- 1 1/2 celery ribs, diced
- 1 1/2 cups soy milk, unsweetened
- 1/4 tsp cayenne pepper
- 1/8 tsp salt
- 1/2 tsp ground black pepper

Directions:

1. Pour the vegetable broth into a saucepan and place over high flame to boil.
2. In the meantime, place a frying pan over medium high flame and heat the olive oil. Once hot, stir in the onion and celery with the salt. Saute for about 3 minutes, or until tender and translucent.
3. Once the vegetable broth is boiling, put the broccoli in it and cook for about 2 minutes or until the pieces become vividly green. Add the spinach and cook for 1 minute or until wilted.
4. Scrape the onion and celery with the olive oil into the saucepan with the broccoli. Remove the saucepan from the heat, then stir in the soy milk and set aside to cool slightly.
5. Put the silken tofu in a bowl and break it up with your hands. Scrape the tofu into the saucepan, then season with salt and

pepper.
6. Using an immersion blender, food processor, or regular blender, blend the slightly cooled soup until all the ingredients are pureed.
7. Return the soup into the saucepan if you didn't use an immersion blender, then place over the medium flame to heat through. Adjust the seasoning, then stir well and serve.

Spinach Pancakes

Ingredients:

- 4 eggs
- 2 cups fresh spinach leaves, chopped
- 1/4 teaspoon salt
- 1 cup flour
- 3/4 cup water
- 1 tsp. olive oil

Directions:

1. Combine egg, flour, water, and salt in a bowl. Mix well until all ingredients are well-combined.
2. Meanwhile, heat the olive oil in a non-stick skillet. Pour batter and mix in the spinach leaves. Cook for 2 minutes or until set. Flip on the other side and cook for another minute.
3. Repeat the same cooking procedure until the rest of the batter is used up.

Baked Omelet with Baby Spinach

Ingredients:

- 6 eggs, whisked until frothy
- 1 white onion, minced
- 2 garlic clove, minced
- 2 cups baby spinach
- 1 Tbsp. pumpkin seeds, roasted
- ½ cup Parmesan cheese, shredded
- ½ Tbsp. olive oil

Directions:

1. Preheat the oven to 375 degrees F. lightly grease cups of muffin tins.
2. Meanwhile, in a skillet, heat the olive oil. Saute garlic and onion for 3 minutes or until limp and translucent. Add in baby spinach and bell peppers. Cook until spinach is wilted. Transfer to a holding plate.
3. Put together eggs and half of Parmesan cheese in a bowl.
4. Put just the right amount of stir-fried vegetables into the muffin cups.
5. Sprinkle pumpkin seeds on top. Pour egg mixture into the cup. Scatter parmesan cheese on top.
6. Place muffin tins into the oven. Bake for 25 minutes or until the eggs are set and the cheese turns golden brown.
7. Remove from the oven. Transfer to a wire rack and let cool for 5 minutes. Extract omelets from the muffin tins. Serve.

Breakfast Pea Soup

Ingredients:

- 1 cup dried green split peas
- 2 garlic cloves
- ½ cup onion, chopped
- ½ cup red bell pepper chopped
- ½ cup celery, chopped
- 2 teaspoons Creole seasoning
- 3 cups vegetable broth, reduced sodium
- 2 cups water
- ½ cup tomato sauce
- 3 tablespoons sour cream, fat free
- 1 tablespoon extra-virgin olive oil

Directions:

1. Heat the olive oil in a saucepan set over medium heat Add in onion, garlic, celery, pepper, and Creole seasoning. Stir well. Cover and cook for 5 minutes or until vegetables are tender.
2. Pour vegetable broth, tomato sauce, and water. Mix well until all ingredients are well combined. Cover and bring to a boil. Reduce the heat. Allow to simmer for 30 minutes or until the peas are tender
3. Transfer 2 cups of the soup into a blender. Tip in garlic cloves. Process until smooth. Return mixture into the saucepan.
4. To serve, garnish with a dollop of sour cream.

Morning Date Muffins

Ingredients:

- 1 cup cashew flour
- 1 tsp baking soda
- 2 Tbsp. coconut flour
- 2 tsp tapioca starch
- 2 cups chia seeds
- 1 1/2 tsp brown sugar
- 2/3 cup ground flax seeds
- 1 tsp cinnamon
- 1 cup diced walnuts
- 2/3 cup applesauce
- 2 cups zucchini, shredded
- 2 cups Medjool dates, chopped
- 3 Tbsp. melted coconut oil, unrefined

Directions:

1. Set the oven to 375°F to preheat. Line 18 muffin tins with paper liners.
2. Put the chia seeds in a bowl and add just enough water to cover them. Set aside to thicken for at least 12 minutes.
3. Meanwhile, combine the flours, flax seeds, baking soda, cinnamon, and tapioca starch in a large bowl.
4. Fold in the walnuts, applesauce, dates, coconut oil, sugar, zucchini, and thickened chia seeds. Mix well.
5. Divide the batter among the prepared muffin tins.
6. Bake for 35 to 40 minutes. Set on a wire rack to cool before serving.

Chapter 7 – Salad recipes

Mixed Salad Greens

Ingredients:

For the salad

- 2 leeks, minced
- 4 cups kale leaves, shredded,
- ½ cup cilantro leaves
- 2 celery stalks, minced
- ½ cup mint leaves
- ½ cup basil leaves
- ½ cup pumpkin seeds, roasted

For the dressing

- 1 banana chili, chopped
- 2 garlic cloves, crushed
- 1 green chili, chopped
- ½ cup lime juice, freshly squeezed
- 1 tablespoon palm sugar, crumbled
- Pinch of salt
- Pinch of pepper

Directions:

1. For the salad, mix kale, leeks, celery, cilantro, basil, and mint leaves. Position the lid and lock in place. Put to high heat and bring to high pressure. Adjust heat to stabilize. Cook for 6 minutes.
2. To make the dressing, combine palm sugar, lime juice, chillies, and garlic cloves. Season with salt and pepper. Stir well until

the sugar and salt dissolve.
3. Remove from heat. Open the pressure cooker. Transfer mixture in a salad dish. Pour the dressing. Sprinkle with pumpkin seeds before serving.

Dark Bulgur Wheat Salad

Ingredients:

- 150g green lentils
- 150g dark bulgur wheat
- 2 ripe tomatoes
- 1 red onion
- 2 garlic cloves
- 2 red peppers
- 2 fresh bay leaves
- 6 spring onions
- 1 teaspoon sumac
- ½ bunch fresh mint
- ½ bunch fresh flat-leaf parsley
- ½ bunch fresh dill
- 2 lemons
- 4 tablespoons pomegranate molasses
- 2 tablespoons extra-virgin olive oil

Directions:

1. Place bulgur in a bowl and add boiling water until just covered. Set aside and leave for 45 minutes.
2. Add bay leaves, garlic, and lentils in the pressure cooker. Pour in cold water until just covered. Position the lid and lock in place. Put to high heat and bring to high pressure. Adjust heat to stabilize. Cook for 5 minutes. Adjust taste if necessary. Drain in a colander. Discard bay leaves and garlic. Transfer lentils in a large bowl.
3. Drain bulgur in a colander then place in a cheesecloth. Squeeze out as much excess water as possible. Add the bulgur

into the bowl with lentils.
4. Trim spring onions and slice. Remove the skin and seeds from the tomatoes and chop. Remove the seeds from the red peppers and slice. Remove the skin from the onion and slice thinly. Roughly chop mint leaves and parsley. Finely chop dill.
5. Add onions, tomatoes, red peppers, onion, mint leaves, parsley, and dill into the bowl with lentils. Add salt and pepper and mix together. Add in the olive oil, lemon zest, pomegranate molasses, and lemon juice. Toss until well-combined.
6. Set aside for 30 minutes. Then, sprinkle with sumac before serving. Serve.

Asparagus and Green Peas Salad

Ingredients:

- 1 cup green peas
- 1 carrot, chopped
- 1 lb. asparagus trimmed
- 1 bunch frisée
- 1 red onion, chopped
- 1 rib celery, chopped
- 1 tablespoon flaxseed oil
- ½ teaspoon Dijon mustard
- 2 tablespoons balsamic vinegar
- 1 tablespoon extra-virgin olive oil
- ½ cup goat cheese, crumbled

Directions:

1. Preheat the oven to 450 degrees F.
2. Pour 3 cups of water to a large saucepan and bring to a boil. Add in onion lentils, carrots, and celery. Reduce heat and allow to simmer for 15 minutes or until the lentils are tender. Drain. Set aside.
3. Meanwhile, layer asparagus on a baking sheet. Tilt sheet to roll asparagus to coat with cooking spray. Roast for 15 minutes.
4. In another bowl, put together mustard and balsamic vinegar. Whisk in flaxseed oil and olive oil. Mix well. Drizzle in lentil mixture. Toss until well coated.
5. To serve, arrange frisée on plates. Put a lentil mixture and sprinkle goat cheese.

Reds Salad on Bacon and Balsamic Vinaigrette

Ingredients:

Red salad

- 1 head red leaf lettuce, torn
- 2 red oak leaf lettuce, torn
- ½ cup radicchio, julienned

Dressing

- 6 streaky bacon
- 2 tablespoons extra virgin olive oil
- ⅛ cup balsamic vinegar
- 2 garlic cloves, grated
- 1 Tbsp. Dijon mustard
- Dash of red pepper flakes
- Pinch of sea salt, add more if needed
- Pinch of black pepper, add more if needed

Directions:

1. For the dressing, pour olive oil into a nonstick skillet. Fry streaky bacon for 3 minutes or until golden brown. Transfer to a plate and crumble into small pieces. Set aside.
2. In the same pan, add in garlic, balsamic vinegar, Dijon mustard, red pepper flakes, salt, and pepper. Whisk until mixture is well blended. Set aside.
3. To assemble, in a big salad bowl, put together red leaf lettuce, red oak leaf lettuce, and radicchio. Drizzle in dressing. Top

with bacon bits. Serve.

Arugula, Lettuce, and Strawberry Salad

Ingredients:

- 12 quail eggs, hardboiled, halved

Salad

- ½ pound romaine lettuce, torn
- 1 pound arugula leaves, torn
- 1 leek, sliced thinly
- 1 cup roasted chicken, cubed
- ½ pound strawberries, quartered
- ¼ cup pine nuts, toasted

Vinaigrette

- ¼ tsp. tomato puree
- 1/3 cup raspberry vinegar
- Pinch of sea salt
- Pinch of black pepper, to taste
- 1/3 cup extra virgin olive oil

Directions:

1. Put together raspberry vinegar, tomato puree, olive oil, salt, and pepper in a mixing bowl. Transfer to a bottle with tight fitting lid. Shake well. Refrigerate for 1 hour or until ready to use.
2. Meanwhile, in a large salad bowl, combine arugula leaves, romaine lettuce, strawberries, leeks, pine nuts, and cubed chicken. Drizzle in half of the vinaigrette. Toss well to

combine. Drizzle in some more of the dressing if desired. Serve.

Curry Tuna Salad

Ingredients:

For the onion pickle

- 1 onion, sliced thinly
- Pinch of sea salt

For the filling

- 4 Romaine lettuce leaves, chilled
- 1 can tuna chunks in water, drained
- 1 Tbsp. Greek yogurt
- 1 Tbsp. tuna brine
- 1 Tbsp. English mustard
- Pinch of sea salt
- Pinch of white pepper
- Dash of Spanish paprika
- Dash of curry powder

Directions:

1. For the onion pickle, mash onion slices using your hands. Season with salt. Set aside, uncovered for 15 minutes.
2. Rinse onions under running water and make sure to drain well. Set aside.
3. For the tuna filling, put together tuna brine, tuna chunks Greek yogurt, Spanish paprika, English mustard, curry powder, salt, white pepper, and green chili in a large bowl. Place inside the fridge to chill for 1 hour or until ready to use.
4. To serve, spread just the right amount of filling along the inner spine of the lettuce leaf. Serve with the onion pickle on the

side.

Beets Cucumber Salad with Curry Vinaigrette

Ingredients:

For the Vinaigrette

- 1 garlic clove, quartered
- 3 Tbsp. curry powder
- 3 Tbsp. lime juice, freshly squeezed
- ¼ cup coconut oil, melted
- Pinch of sea salt, add more if needed
- Pinch of black pepper, to taste
- 3 Tbsp. coconut vinegar

Salad

- 2 cucumbers, processed into flat noodles
- 1 cup baby beet greens
- 2 parsley, minced, for garnish
- 2 pears, quartered, sliced thinly

Directions:

1. Put together garlic clove, curry powder, lime juice, coconut vinegar, coconut oil, salt, and pepper in a small mixing bowl. Stir well.
2. Transfer vinaigrette to a bottle with tight fitting lid. Shake.
3. Meanwhile, put baby beet greens, spiralized cucumbers, pears, and parsley in a salad bowl. Drizzle in an equal amount of vinaigrette. Serve.

Roasted Carrots and Cashew Salad on Lemon Vinaigrette

Ingredients:
  Roasted carrots

- 2 carrots, cubed
- ½ cup cashew nuts, halved
- 2 tsp. cumin powder
- Pinch of sea salt
- Pinch of black pepper, to taste
- ½ Tbsp. olive oil

For the lemon vinaigrette

- 1 tsp. extra virgin olive oil
- 1 lemon, juiced
- 1 Tbsp. stevia
- Pinch of sea salt
- Pinch of black pepper

For the salad greens

- 2 bags arugula, chopped
- 2 bags baby spinach, chopped

Directions:

1. Preheat the oven to 400 degrees F. Line a baking sheet with parchment paper.
2. Put together olive oil, carrots, cumin powder, and cashew nuts in a bowl. Season with salt and pepper.

3. Place mixture onto the baking sheet. Roast for 30 minutes.
4. Remove from the oven and allow to cool for few minutes.
5. To make the lemon vinaigrette, combine lemon juice, olive oil, salt, pepper, and stevia in a separate bowl.
6. Drizzle in dressing over cooked carrots. Set aside.
7. Put together arugula, baby spinach, and roasted veggies in a salad bowl. Toss well to combine.
8. To serve, drizzle in just the right amo8unt of vinaigrette over salad.

Baby Spinach, Chicken, and Carrot Salad with Peanut Butter Dressing

Ingredients:

- 3 cups baby spinach
- 2 cups chicken breast, boneless, skinless cooked, thinly sliced
- ½ cup scallions, sliced
- 1 garlic clove, crushed
- 2 cups baby peas
- ½ cup carrot, shredded
- ½ teaspoon ginger, grated
- 1 tablespoon flaxseed oil
- 1 teaspoon sesame oil
- 2 teaspoons soy sauce, low sodium
- 2 tablespoons natural peanut butter
- ¼ cup warm water
- Fresh cilantro, for garnish

Directions:

1. Place an equal amount of baby spinach on plates. Fan chicken slices over the spinach. Sprinkle scallions, peas, and carrots.
2. In a small bowl, whisk together flaxseed oil, sesame oil, peanut butter, and soy sauce. Mix until smooth. Pour warm water. Tip in ginger and garlic.
3. Drizzle dressing over the salad. Garnish with cilantro.

Radicchio, Watercress, and Pecans Salad with Red Wine Dressing

Ingredients

- 3 heads radicchio
- 3 bunches watercress
- 1 oz. dried cranberries
- 2 oz. toasted pecans
- 3 bulbs fennel
- 3 cloves garlic
- 2 tbsp. red wine vinegar
- 2 tbsp. balsamic vinegar
- 225 ml. extra virgin olive oil

Directions

1. In a small bowl, combine the red wine vinegar, garlic, cranberries, and balsamic vinegar.
2. Slowly whisk in the olive oil to emulsify.
3. In a large salad bowl, combine the radicchio, watercress, fennel and pecans.
4. Pour the balsamic dressing over salad; toss well and serve.

Plum Tomatoes and Peppers Salad

Ingredients:

- 8 plum tomatoes
- 4 yellow peppers
- 4 long red peppers
- 1 tablespoon baby capers
- 2 large red onions
- 6 garlic cloves
- 1 teaspoon paprika
- ½ lemon
- 4 tablespoons extra-virgin olive oil

Directions:

1. Slice tomatoes in half and cut the onions into quarters. Place tomatoes and onions inside the pressure cooker. Tip in red and yellow peppers and garlic.
2. Drizzle oil all over the vegetables and season with salt. Position the lid and lock in place. Put to high heat and bring to high pressure. Adjust heat to stabilize. Cook for 5 minutes.
3. Place the peppers on a chopping board and immediately remove the skin and seeds. Cut into strips then place on a bowl.
4. Add the onion and tomatoes into the bowl. Remove the tough skins from the garlic and add into the bowl.
5. Add the paprika, capers, lemon juice, and 4 tablespoons of extra-virgin olive oil into the bowl. Season with black pepper and sea salt and mix together using hands. Serve warm or cold with a fresh drizzle of olive oil.

Spinach and Avocado with Quail Eggs

Ingredients:

Salad

- 2 baby spinach leaves
- Pinch of sea salt
- Pinch of black pepper
- 1 Tbsp. balsamic vinegar
- 1 tsp. extra virgin olive oil

- ½ avocado, diced
- 4 asparagus, sliced into long slivers
- 8 quail eggs
- Parmesan cheese, for garnish

Directions:

1. Preheat the oven to 400 degrees °F. Lightly grease laminated paper liners into a muffin tin.
2. Put diced avocadoes into paper lines and top with asparagus slivers. Crack open 2 quail eggs into each muffin cup. Season with salt.
3. Transfer muffin tin into the oven and bake for 15 minutes or until eggs are set. Remove from heat.
4. Allow to cool on a cake rack before removing paper liners.
5. To serve, put together spinach leaves, balsamic vinegar, salt, pepper and olive oil in a salad bowl. Put the baked quail eggs. Sprinkle Parmesan cheese. Serve.

Eggplant and Pine Nuts Salad

Ingredients:

- 4 small eggplant, sliced lengthwise
- 1 tablespoon toasted pine nuts
- 1 shallot, thinly sliced
- ¼ teaspoon fine sea salt
- 2 tablespoons basil leaves, chopped
- 2 tablespoons lemon juice, freshly squeezed
- ½ tablespoon extra-virgin olive oil

Directions:

1. Set the grill to medium high heat. Grill eggplant for 5 minutes on each side.
2. Meanwhile, in a bowl, combine lemon juice, oil, shallot, and salt. Mix until well combined.
3. Chop eggplant. Add to the dressing. Toss to combine. Fold in pine nuts and basil. Serve.

Ripe Tomatoes and Basil Salad

Ingredients:

- 1½ pounds ripe tomatoes, sliced into thick medallions
- 1 handful basil leaves, julienned
- 1½ pounds mozzarella, sliced thinly
- Pinch of sea salt
- Pinch of black pepper
- extra virgin olive oil, for drizzling

Directions:

1. Using a serving platter, layer tomatoes and mozzarella slices. Sprinkle basil leaves. Season with salt and black pepper. Drizzle in olive oil.
2. Place inside the refrigerator to chill for 1 hour or until ready to serve.

Mango, Kiwi, and Berries Salad

Ingredients:

- 1 mango, ripe, cubed
- 1 kiwi fruit, quartered
- ½ cup blueberries
- 1 strawberry, quartered

For the Dressing

- ⅛ teaspoon maple syrup
- 1 tablespoon lime juice, freshly squeezed
- Pinch of sea salt

Directions:

1. To make the dressing, pour lime juice, maple syrup, and salt into a bottle with tight fitting lid. Seal. Shake well.
2. Put mango, kiwi, blueberries, and strawberry into a large salad bowl. Drizzle in just the right amount of dressing. Toss well to combine. Serve.

Bulgur, Cucumber, and Orange Salad

Ingredients:

- 1 cup bulgur wheat
- ½ cucumber, diced
- 2 oranges, seedless, cut into segments
- 2 cups water
- 1 green pepper, diced
- 1 lemon rind, grated
- 4 tablespoons almonds, roasted
- 1 lemon, freshly squeezed
- ½ cup fresh mint, chopped
- Pinch of salt
- Pinch of ground black pepper
- Fresh mint sprigs, to garnish

Directions:

1. Put together water and bulgur wheat in a bowl. Set aside for 20 minutes.
2. Drain soaked bulgur wheat using a colander. Squeeze out as much liquid. Transfer to a bowl.
3. Add green pepper, cucumber, lemon rind, mint, and toasted almonds. Put lemon juice. Mix well.
4. Add orange segments and juice into the bulgur mixture. Season with salt and pepper. Mix. Garnish with mint sprigs.

Cucumber, Lettuce, and Crab Meat Salad

Ingredients:

Salad

- 2 cucumber, sliced into thick matchsticks
- 2 heads Romaine lettuce, shredded
- 1 tub crab meat, shredded

Dressing

- 1 teaspoon ginger, grated
- ¼ teaspoon fish sauce
- 1 teaspoon palm sugar, crumbled
- 1 tablespoon light soy sauce
- 1 tablespoon rice wine vinegar
- Pinch of sea salt
- Pinch of black pepper
- ¼ cup extra virgin olive oil

Directions:

1. Pour dressing ingredients in a small container with tight fitting lid; shake well to combine. Taste; adjust seasoning if needed. Set aside.
2. Place salad ingredients in mixing bowl; drizzle in half of dressing. Toss to combine; spoon equal portions of salad into plates. Drizzle in remaining dressing. Serve.

Creamy Chicken, Grapes, and Chestnuts Salad

Ingredients:

- 3 cups salad greens
- 1 ½ cup chicken, cooked, chopped
- 1 orange, sliced
- ½ cup celery, chopped
- 1/3 cup grapes, sliced
- 1 green onion, chopped
- 4 oz water chestnuts, sliced
- 3 oz nonfat yogurt
- 1 tablespoon light soy sauce

Directions:

1. Combine the soy sauce and yogurt in a bowl. Set aside.
2. Toss the remaining ingredients, except salad greens, in a bowl. Add the dressing and toss well.
3. Chill the mixture for 2 hours, then spoon over the salad greens.

Beans Salad

Ingredients:

- 7.5 oz canned black beans, drained
- 7.5 oz canned cannellini beans, drained
- 1 avocado, diced
- ½ red onion, diced
- ½ jalapeno pepper, minced
- 1 yellow bell pepper, diced
- 2 tablespoons fresh cilantro, chopped
- 1/3 cup tomatillo salsa, low sodium
- Pinch of sea salt

Directions:

1. Combine the bell pepper, cilantro, beans, onion, and jalapeno in a bowl.
2. Fold in the salsa and avocado. Season with salt and serve.

Tofu and Broccoli Salad

Ingredients:

- 1 lb tofu, cubed
- 1 onion, sliced
- 1 cup broccoli, divided into florets
- 2 red bell peppers, sliced
- 2 tablespoons olive oil
- 1 tablespoon sesame oil
- 1 garlic clove, crushed
- 1 carrot, julienne strips
- 1 stick celery, sliced
- 1 tablespoon tamarind concentrate
- 1 tablespoon tomato puree
- 2 tablespoons oyster sauce
- 1 tablespoon light soy sauce
- 1 tablespoon chilli sauce
- 1 tablespoon fish sauce
- Pinch of ground star anise
- 8 oz mangetout snow peas, halved
- 4 oz thin French beans, halved
- 2 tablespoons sugar
- 1 teaspoon cornflour
- 2 cups water
- 1 tablespoon white wine vinegar

Directions:

1. In a wok, heat the oil. Add garlic and cook for 2 minutes.

2. Add tofu in batches or until golden brown on all sides. Remove and set aside.
3. Add onion, red bell pepper, celery, carrots, snow peas, green beans, and broccoli for 3 minutes or until tender crisp.
4. Add oyster sauce, fish sauce, chilli sauce, vinegar, tomato puree, sugar, and star anise in a bowl. Mix well.
5. Mix the cornflour with water. Add to the tofu. Stir fry until the sauce boils and thickens. Serve.

Chapter 8 – Lunch Recipes

Beef Chili and Beans

Ingredients:

- 1 can kidney beans
- 1 can pinto beans
- 1 lb. lean ground beef
- 1 onion, minced
- 2 garlic, grated
- 2 cans diced tomatoes
- 1 cup beef stock
- 1 Tbsp. hot pepper sauce
- 1 tsp. tomato paste
- 1 green chili pepper, minced
- 2 Tbsp. chili powder
- 1 Tbsp. cumin powder
- ¼ tsp. sugar
- 1 tsp. sea salt
- 1 tsp. black pepper
- ¼ cup fresh parsley, minced, for garnish

Directions:

1. Place ground beef into large Dutch oven set over high heat. Stir-fry to brown meat, breaking up larger clumps as you go. Drain excess grease, if any.
2. Except for parsley, add in remaining ingredients into Dutch oven. Stir. Season lightly. Let chili come to a boil. Put lid on. Turn down heat to lowest setting. Let chili simmer for 30 minutes to fully cook meat, and soften onions. Turn off heat.
3. Ladle chili into individual portions. Garnish with minced parsley, if using. Cool slightly before serving.

Pumpkin and Apples Soup

Ingredients

- 1 pumpkin
- 2 carrots, chopped
- 1 green apple, sliced
- 4 celery stalks, chopped
- 1 yellow onion, chopped
- 3 cups vegetable stock
- 1 tsp. chili powder
- 2 tbsp. ghee
- 1/2 tsp. cumin powder
- 2 tsp. cinnamon powder
- 1 1/2 tsp. sea salt
- 3 tbsp. olive oil

Directions:

1. Pre-heat the oven to about 400 degrees F.
2. In a large bowl, combine the butternut squash, 1/2 tsp. salt, 1 tsp. cinnamon, olive oil, and 1/2 tsp. cumin.
3. Coat the pumpkin and mix together; spread mixture on a rimmed baking sheet.
4. Toss the onion, apple slices, celery stalks and carrots to coat.
5. Place on a rimmed baking sheet and roast 40 minutes, until soft.
6. In a large pot, heat the ghee, add the roasted ingredients, vegetable broth, and add 1 teaspoon each of chili powder, salt and cinnamon.
7. Bring it to a boil, reduce the heat and simmer for 20 minutes.
8. In a food processor, blend the ingredients until smooth; serve

warm.

9. If you want to spice up this recipe, add 2 chipotle chilies (adobo sauce) to replace the chili powder.

Tuna Fillets with All Tomatoes Salad

Ingredients:

For the Fish fillets

- 8 tuna fillets
- 1 tsp. red pepper flakes
- 2 Tbsp. Spanish paprika powder
- 1 lime, sliced into wedges
- ½ tsp. sea salt
- olive oil

For the Tomato Salad

- 2 beefsteak tomatoes, unripe, cubed
- 2 red salad tomatoes, ripe, cubed
- ¼ lb. cherry tomatoes, quartered
- 1 leek, minced
- fresh cilantro, minced
- 1 Tbsp. balsamic vinegar
- Pinch of sea salt
- Pinch of black pepper

Directions:

1. For the tomato salad, put together red salad tomatoes, cherry tomatoes, beefsteak tomatoes, balsamic vinegar, salt, pepper, leek and cilantro in a lidded, non-reactive container. Toss all ingredients until well-combined. Place inside the fridge to chill until ready to serve.
2. For the tuna grill, set the grill pan to medium heat. Lightly grease the grill surface with olive oil.

3. Put together red pepper flakes, Spanish paprika, and salt in a bowl. Use the mixture to rub all sides of the fish fillets. Grill for 5 minutes on one side. Flip to the other side and grill for 3 minutes.
4. Transfer to a holding plate. Cover fish with aluminum foil. Let sit for 5 minutes.
5. To serve, place one tuna fillet on a plate. Put just the right amount of tomato salad. Squeeze lime juice all over.

Cauliflower, Carrots, and Peas Curry

Ingredients:

- 3 cups cauliflower florets, chopped into bite-sized pieces
- 1 cup green peas
- ½ cup carrot, chopped
- 2 teaspoons garlic, minced
- ½ cup onion, chopped
- 1 ½ cups vegetable broth
- 1 teaspoon curry powder
- Pinch of salt
- 3 teaspoons olive oil, divided
- ½ cup plain yogurt, fat free
- Fresh cilantro leaves, for garnish

Directions:

1. Heat the olive oil in a deep skillet set over medium heat. Once the oil is hot, add in cauliflower florets. Cover, whilst tossing occasionally for 5 minutes. Transfer to a plate and set aside.
2. Add remaining olive oil and saute onions, garlic, carrots, and brown lentils Season with curry powder. Stir mixture and cook for 3 minutes.
3. Pour vegetable broth. Bring mixture to a boil. Reduce the heat and a low mixture to simmer for 20 minutes.
4. Tip in cooked cauliflower into the skillet and cook, partially covered for 5 minutes. Season with salt. Adjust taste as needed.
5. To serve, spoon an equal amount into plates. Dollop on yogurt. Garnish with cilantro.

Halibut with Orange and Broccoli

Ingredients:

- 4 halibut fillets, boneless, skinless
- 3 cups broccoli florets
- 2 navel oranges
- 3 teaspoons olive oil
- 1 cup red onions, cut half crosswise
- Pinch of salt, add more if needed
- 3 teaspoons orange zest, grated, divided
- 2 tablespoons water
- Pinch of ground black pepper

Directions:

1. Preheat the oven to 375 degrees F. Line a baking sheet with aluminum foil. Lightly coat with cooking spray.
2. Place onions, cut side down on a pan. Break slices into separate pieces and transfer to the baking sheet
3. Drizzle in olive oil and sprinkle salt. Layer and spread onions evenly on the baking sheet.
4. Roast for 20 minutes or until the onions are golden.
5. Remove baking sheet from the oven and add the oranges. Toss well to coat. Return to the oven and roast for 5 minutes.
6. Remove from the baking sheet and spread onion mixture into a platter. Lay halibut fillets on top. Drizzle in orange zest. Return to the oven and roast for 10 minutes.
7. In a skillet, put together olive oil and water. Bring mixture to a boil. Add in broccoli. Season with salt. Cook for 5 minutes.
8. To serve, divide onion mixture to plates and top with halibut, and broccoli. Drizzle in remaining orange zest.

Chicken Fillet Soup

Ingredients:

- 2 pounds chicken thigh fillets
- 1 thumb-sized ginger, crushed
- 2 garlic cloves, minced
- 2 onions, minced
- 2 Tbsp. fish sauce
- 2 unripe papaya, cubed
- 4 cups water
- Pinch of sea salt
- Pinch of black pepper
- ½ cup chili leaves, rinsed
- 2 Tbsp. olive oil, divided

Directions:

1. Pour olive oil into a Dutch oven. Fry chicken thigh fillets, in batches, for 5 minutes or until golden brown. Transfer to a plate.
2. Pour the remaining olive oil. Saute onion, garlic, and ginger for 3 minutes or until limp.
3. Add in cooked chicken fillets, papaya, water, fish sauce, salt, and pepper. Bring mixture to a boil. Reduce heat and bring to a simmer for 10 minutes or until the chicken is tender. Add in chili leaves.
4. To serve, ladle soup and chicken into bowls.

Mackerel Steaks in Butter

Ingredients:

- 2 Tbsp. butter, divided
- 4 Spanish mackerel steaks
- ¼ cup garlic, grated
- Pinch of sea salt to taste
- 2 Tbsp. olive oil

Directions:

1. Season Spanish mackerel steaks with just small amount of salt. Set aside.
2. Meanwhile heat the olive oil in a non-stick skillet. Saute garlic for 3 minutes or until golden. Set aside.
3. Add in half of the butter into the same skillet. Fry mackerel steaks for 4 minutes. Set aside.
4. Add in remaining butter. Cook fish thoroughly for 5 minutes. Garnish with garlic on top. Serve.

Tart Apple and Carrots Soup

Ingredients:

- 2 tart apples, chopped
- 8 carrots, sliced
- 1 celery rib, sliced
- 1 onion, chopped
- 1 tbsp. ghee
- 1/2 tsp. sage
- 1/4 tsp. pepper
- 5 cups vegetable stock
- 1 bay leaf

Directions:

1. In a pan, cook carrots, onions, apples, and celery with ghee; stir until fruits and vegetables turn tender.
2. Add the pepper, vegetable broth, bay leaf and safe.
3. Bring to a rolling bowl until carrots turns tender.
4. Transfer contents into a food processor; blend until smooth.
5. Pour contents into the same pan and heat until ready to serve in bowls.

Black Bean and Avocado Soup

Ingredients:

- 8 oz canned black beans
- 1/2 small avocado
- 2 garlic cloves, minced
- 1/2 red onion, minced
- 1 1/2 cups vegetable stock
- 1 red bell pepper, diced
- 1/2 tbsp. dried oregano
- 1/2 tbsp. ground cumin
- 1/8 tsp ground turmeric
- 3/4 tsp paprika
- 1/4 tsp red pepper flakes
- 1/4 tsp sea salt
- 1/4 tsp ground black pepper
- 1 tbsp. lime juice, freshly squeezed
- 1/2 bay leaf
- tbsp. olive oil

Directions:

1. Drain the canned black beans thoroughly, then transfer into a colander and rinse under cold running water. Set aside to drain.
2. Place a soup pot over medium flame and add the canola oil. Once hot, stir in the garlic and saute until you can sniff the aroma, which will take about half a minute.
3. Stir in the onion and some of the salt. Saute until the onion becomes tender, then stir in the red bell pepper and saute until bell pepper is tender.

4. Add the broth into the pot, then stir in the black beans, bay leaf, lime juice, black pepper, cumin, oregano, paprika, red pepper flakes, and turmeric.
5. Stir in the remaining salt, then cover the pot and allow the soup to simmer for about 20 minutes. Fish out the bay leaf and discard.
6. If desired, you can pour half of the soup into a blender or a food processor, or use an immersion blender to puree the mixture. Reheat the soup afterwards if you have decided to go through this step.
7. Ladle the soup into three bowls, then slice the avocado into cubes and divide the cubes among the three servings. Serve at once.

Bulgur Chili with Tomatoes and Beans

Ingredients:

- ½ cup bulgur
- 1 onion, minced
- 3 garlic clove, minced
- 1 carrot, minced
- 2 jalapeño peppers, minced
- 2 cans diced tomatoes
- 1 can black beans
- 1 can cannelloni beans
- 2 tsp. cayenne pepper
- 1 tsp. ground cumin
- ½ tsp. tomato paste
- 2 cups mushroom stock
- Pinch of salt
- ¼ cup fresh cilantro, minced, for garnish
- ¼ tsp. olive oil

Directions:

1. Pour oil into large Dutch oven set over high heat. Sauté garlic, onion and *jalapeño* pepper, until onion is limp and transparent, about 1 minute.
2. Except for cilantro, add in remaining ingredients. Stir. Put lid on. Cook chili for 45 to 50 minutes, stirring often. Taste. Adjust seasoning according.
3. Ladle chili into individual portions. Garnish with fresh cilantro, if desired. Serve warm.

Zucchini and Shrimps Salad

Ingredients:

- 1 pound shrimps, deveined
- Pinch of sea salt
- Pinch of black pepper
- ½ pound fresh kale leaves, shredded
- ¾ tablespoon five-spice powder
- 3 tablespoons olive oil

Salad

- 1 zucchini, processed into spaghetti noodles
- 1 white onion, julienned
- 1 carrot, julienned
- 1 ginger, julienned
- 3 tablespoons sesame oil
- ¼ cup rice wine vinegar
- 1 lime, sliced into wedges

Directions:

1. Pour 2 tablespoons of olive oil into wok set over high heat. Sauté shrimps with salt, five spice powder and pepper; cook until shrimps turn coral. Transfer cooked pieces into salad bowl.
2. Pour remaining olive oil into same wok; add in kale leaves and small pinch of salt. Cook until leaves wilt. Place kale leaves on top of shrimps; cool before adding in remaining ingredients.
3. Place remaining ingredients into salad bowl. Toss well to combine; spoon equal portions into plates. Taste; adjust

seasoning if needed. Serve.

Creamy and Cheesy Aubergine

Ingredients:

- 1 aubergine, sliced into thick medallions
- 1 tablespoon butter
- 1 tablespoon cream cheese
- ½ cup milk, low fat
- 1 tablespoon almond flour, finely milled
- ¼ cup cheddar cheese, grated
- ¼ cup gouda cheese, smoked, grated
- Pinch of black pepper
- olive oil, for greasing

Directions:

1. Preheat the oven to 400°F. Line a baking sheet with aluminum foil. Lightly grease with oil. Layer aubergine on top.
2. Meanwhile, put butter and almond flour in saucepan. Whisk well until flour clumps together. Pour milk. Season with pepper. Mix.
3. Add in cheddar cheese and gouda cheese. Stir until the mixture is smooth and creamy. Remove from heat.
4. Transfer to a serving plate. Serve.

Pressure Cooked Mixed Vegetables

Ingredients:

- 1 broccoli, sliced into bite-sized florets, stem sliced into thick matchsticks
- 1 ginger, julienned
- 1 shallot, julienned
- 2 garlic cloves, minced
- 1 carrot, sliced into ⅛-inch thick matchsticks
- 1 Tbsp. coconut oil
- 1 cup snow peas
- Pinch of kosher salt
- Pinch of white pepper, to taste
- 2 Tbsp. mushroom stock

Directions:

1. Pour oil into the pressure cooker. Add in and sauté garlic cloves, ginger and shallot until limp and aromatic. Pour in mushroom stock. Add in broccoli and carrots.
2. Position the lid and lock in place. Put to high heat and bring to high pressure. Adjust heat to stabilize. Cook for 5 minutes.
3. Add in snow peas. Reposition the lid and lock in place. Put to high heat and bring to high pressure. Adjust heat to stabilize. Cook for another 3 minutes.
4. Taste and season dish lightly. Divide into equal portions. Serve.

Cauliflower, Spinach, and Garbanzo Beans Curry

Ingredients:

- 4 cups fresh spinach, chopped
- 1 cup cauliflower florets, chopped
- 1 cup garbanzo beans, cooked
- 12 oz canned diced tomatoes
- 1 tsp whole mustard seeds
- 1 yellow onion, diced
- 2 garlic cloves, minced
- 1 Tbsp. ginger, minced
- 1/4 tsp garlic powder
- 1/2 tsp ground coriander
- 1 1/2 tsp curry powder
- 1 1/2 tsp cumin seeds
- 1/4 tsp ground cinnamon
- 1/16 tsp ground cloves
- 1 tsp sea salt
- 1 green cardamom pod
- 2 Tbsp. coconut oil

Directions:

1. Place a soup pot over medium flame and heat up. Add the oil and mustard seeds. Stir until seeds begin to pop.
2. Stir in the onion and saute until browning. Stir in the garlic, ginger, and 1/2 teaspoon of salt. Mix well and cook for 3 minutes.
3. Stir in the garlic powder, curry powder, coriander, cinnamon, cumin seeds, cloves, cardamom pod, and asafetida. Stir in the

tomatoes with their juices. Let the mixture simmer.
4. Stir in the spinach and cook until wilted. Stir in the cauliflower and garbanzo beans. Add the remaining salt and mix well.
5. Cover, set flame to low, then cook for 20 minutes.
6. Discard out the cardamom pod. Serve.

Chicken and Mushrooms with Zucchini Noodle Soup

Ingredients:

- 1 zucchini, processed into spaghetti-like noodles
- 3 garlic cloves, minced
- 2 white onions, thinly sliced
- 1 thumb-sized ginger, julienned
- 1 lb. chicken thighs
- 1 lb. portabella mushrooms, sliced into thick slivers
- 2 cups chicken stock
- 3 cups water
- Pinch of sea salt, add more if needed
- Pinch of black pepper, add more if needed
- 2 tsp. sesame oil
- 4 Tbsp. coconut oil, divided
- ¼ cup fresh chives, minced, for garnish

Directions:

1. Pour 2 tablespoons of coconut oil into a large saucepan. Fry mushroom slivers in batches for 5 minutes or until seared brown. Set aside. Transfer these to a plate.
2. Saute onion, garlic, and ginger for 3 minutes or until tender. Add in chicken thighs, cooked mushrooms, chicken stock, water, salt, and pepper stir mixture well. Bring to a boil.
3. Reduce heat and allow to simmer for 20 minutes or until the chicken is fork tender. Tip in sesame oil.
4. Serve by placing an equal amount of zucchini noodles into bowls. Ladle soup and garnish with chives.

Tofu Kebabs

Ingredients:

- 28 oz extra firm tofu
- ½ tsp Sriracha sauce
- ½ tsp ginger root, minced
- 1 onion, sliced into wedges
- 6 cherry tomatoes
- 1 Tbsp. tamari sauce
- ½ Tbsp. lime juice, freshly squeezed
- 8 fresh mint leaves
- ½ Tbsp. hoisin sauce
- Coconut oil

Directions:

1. Slice the tofu into large cubes and place between two sheets of paper towels. Press gently with a flat plate until most of the water is squeezed out.
2. Combine the tamari or soy sauce with the lime juice, Sriracha sauce, and ginger. Mix well.
3. Place tofu cubes into the marinade and turn several times to coat. Cover and refrigerate for at least half an hour to marinate.
4. Once the marinated tofu cubes are ready, skewer them with the onion, cherry tomato, and mint leaf until you have six kebabs.
5. Position the lid and lock in place. Put to high heat and bring to high pressure. Adjust heat to stabilize. Cook for 3 minutes.
6. Transfer to a grill pan over medium high flame and heat through. Once hot, coat with coconut oil.

7. Grill the kebabs for about 3 minutes, turning occasionally.
8. Brush kebabs with the hoisin sauce and grill for an additional 3 minutes, turning occasionally. Transfer to a serving dish and serve right away.

Ginger Chicken with Beans and Peas

Ingredients:

- ½ pounds chicken breast fillets, sliced into thick matchsticks
- 1 teaspoon sugar
- 1 teaspoon rice vinegar
- 1 tablespoon light soy sauce

- 1 shallot, minced
- 2 garlic, minced
- 1 ginger, sliced thinly
- 1 pound French beans
- 1 pound snow peas
- ½ cup sesame seeds, toasted
- 3 tablespoons water
- 2 tablespoons peanut oil
- 1 tablespoon cornstarch
- ¼ cup chicken stock
- Pinch of sea salt
- Pinch of black pepper

Directions:

1. Place chicken and marinade in food-safe bag; seal. Massage contents of bag to combine. Marinate in fridge for at least 30 minutes prior to use (or up to 42 hours beforehand.) Drain; reserve marinade. Dissolve cornstarch in water and leftover marinade to make cornstarch slurry. Set aside.

2. Pour ½ tablespoon of peanut oil into non-stick wok set over medium heat; stir-fry half of marinated chicken until seared brown on all sides. Temporarily transfer cooked pieces to a plate. Repeat step for remaining chicken.
3. Pour remaining peanut oil into the same wok; sauté garlic and shallot until limp and aromatic. Return chicken to wok, plus ginger and stock. Stir. Reduce heat to lowest setting. Put lid on; cook chicken for 5 or 7 minutes, or until liquid is slightly reduced.
4. Except for sesame seeds and slurry, add in remaining ingredients into wok; stir-fry until snow peas turn a shade brighter, about 3 to 5 minutes. Pour in cornstarch slurry; cook until sauce thickens. Turn off heat. Taste; adjust seasoning if needed. Spoon equal portions of dish into plates; sprinkle sesame seeds on top. Serve.

Stir-fry veggies with Shrimp and Pork

Ingredients:

- 1 lb. pork belly with rind, sliced into thick pieces
- 1 lb. prawns, peeled, deveined
- ⅛ cup garlic, minced
- 2 onions, minced
- 2 tomatoes, minced
- 1 eggplant, sliced
- ¾ cup water
- 2 banana chili, deseeded

- 1 bitter gourd, sliced
- 1 Tbsp. shrimp paste
- ½ lb. okra, halved
- ¼ lb. string beans, sliced into long slivers
- ½ cup pumpkin, cubed
- 1 Tbsp. coconut vinegar
- 1 Tbsp. coconut oil

Directions:

1. Place pork belly, coconut oil, and water into a large saucepan. Cook for 15 minutes or until the water evaporates and the fat renders out. Reduce heat and cover the lid. Continue cooking until pork belly crisps. Set aside.
2. Sauté garlic for 2 minutes. Do not burn. Add in onion and tomato. Cook for 3 minutes.
3. Tip in okra, string beans, eggplant, and bitter gourd. Cook for 3 minutes.
4. Add Japanese pumpkin, vinegar, shrimp paste, and water.

Secure the lid. Cook for 5 minutes or until pumpkin is tender.
5. Add prawns. Cook liquid is greatly reduced. Season with salt and pepper.
6. Transfer to a platter. Garnish with pork bits.

All Tomatoes Soup with Barley

Ingredients:

- 14 oz canned crushed tomatoes, unsalted
- 1/3 cup tomatoes, sun-dried, chopped
- 14 oz canned tomatoes, fire-roasted
- 1/2 cup pearl barley
- 8 oz canned navy beans, unsalted, drained
- 1 tbsp. herbes de Provence
- 1/4 yellow onion, minced
- 2 garlic cloves, minced
- 1/2 cup almond milk
- 1 cup vegetable stock
- 1/2 tbsp. water
- 1 tsp maple syrup
- 1/2 tbsp. all-purpose or almond flour
- 1/2 tbsp. dried rosemary
- 1/8 tsp crushed red pepper
- 1/8 tsp ground black pepper
- 1/8 tsp white pepper
- 2 tbsp. olive oil

Directions:

1. Place a saucepan over medium flame and heat the olive oil. Stir in the garlic and saute until aromatic. Stir in the onion and saute until soft and translucent.
2. Stir in the sun-dried tomatoes and saute until tender, which will take about 3 minutes.
3. Meanwhile, combine the water and flour in a bowl.
4. Stir into the saucepan along with the remaining tomatoes,

followed by the milk and broth, spices, barley, beans, and maple syrup.
5. Stir the mixture to combine, adjusting the seasoning, if needed. Cover and set to low flame. Let simmer for 20 minutes, or until the barley becomes puffed. Serve at once.

Chili and Beans Quinoa

Ingredients:

- 1/2 cup quinoa, rinsed
- 2 garlic cloves, minced
- 1 onion, diced
- 1/2 red pepper, diced
- 14 oz kidney beans
- 7.5 oz black beans
- 1 cup corn kernels
- 1/2 tsp coriander
- 1 tsp chili powder
- 2 tsp cumin
- 1 1/2 tsp oregano
- 1/2 cup water
- 14 oz diced tomatoes
- 1/2 Tbsp. olive oil

Directions:

1. Combine all of the ingredients in a slow cooker.
2. Cover and cook on low for 6 hours. Serve hot with vegan flat bread or cooked brown rice.

Chapter 8 – Dinner Recipes

No-Bread Beef Bacon Burger

Ingredients:

- 1½ ground beef
- 4 streaky bacon strips, halved
- 2 onions, minced

- olive oil for greasing
- 2 tomatoes, sliced into disks
- 1 zucchini, sliced into disks
- Dash of oregano powder
- Pinch of sea salt
- Pinch of white pepper

Directions:

1. In a big mixing bowl, combine ground beef, onions white pepper, and oregano powder. Mix well. Shape mixture into patties. Sprinkle salt. Set aside.
2. In a nonstick skillet, pour olive oil. Fry bacon strips for 4 minutes or until golden brown. Drain on paper towels. Set aside.
3. Fry patties, flip once, until meat is cooked through. Set aside.
4. Fry tomato medallions until lightly seared. Do the same thing for the zucchini medallions. Season with salt.
5. To serve, stack burgers with tomato, zucchini, beef patty, and bacon slices. Serve.

Grilled Tempeh with Pineapple

Ingredients:

- 10 oz tempeh, sliced
- 1 red bell pepper, quartered
- 1/4 pineapple, sliced into rings
- 6 oz green beans
- 1 tbsp. coconut aminos
- 2 1/2 tbsp. orange juice, freshly squeeze
- 1 1/2 tbsp. lemon juice, freshly squeezed
- 1 tbsp. extra virgin olive oil
- 1/4 cup hoisin sauce

Directions:

1. Mix together the olive oil, orange and lemon juices, coconut aminos or soy sauce, and hoisin sauce in a bowl. Add the diced tempeh and set aside.
2. Preheat the grill or place a grill pan over medium high flame. Once hot, lift the marinated tempeh from the bowl with a pair of tongs and transfer them to the grill or pan.
3. Grill for 2 to 3 minutes, or until browned all over.
4. Grill the sliced pineapples alongside the tempeh, then transfer them directly onto the serving platter.
5. Place the grilled tempeh beside the grilled pineapple and cover with aluminum foil to keep warm.
6. Meanwhile, place the green beans and bell peppers in a bowl and add just enough of the marinade to coat.
7. Prepare the grill pan and add the vegetables. Grill until fork tender and slightly charred.
8. Transfer the grilled vegetables to the serving platter and

arrange artfully with the tempeh and pineapple. Serve at once.

Mushrooms, Chicken, and Chestnuts in Lettuce Wraps

Ingredients:

For the filling

- 1 onion, minced
- 1 tsp. ginger, grated
- 1 garlic clove, minced
- ¾ pound lean ground chicken
- 1 carrot, julienned
- 2 fresh Portabella mushrooms, thinly sliced
- 1 Tbsp. white vinegar
- 1 Tbsp. catsup
- 1 can chestnuts, minced
- 1 tsp. sesame oil
- 1 Tbsp. olive oil

––––––––

- 8 iceberg lettuce leaves, chilled

Directions:

1. Pour olive oil into a non-stick skillet. Add in Portabella mushrooms. Cook for 3 minutes or until brown on both sides. Set aside.
2. In the same skillet, saute onion and garlic for 3 minutes or until fragrant and translucent. Stir in ground chicken. Cook for 4 minutes or until the meat is no longer pink.
3. Stir in ginger, carrot, white vinegar, catsup, and chestnuts into

the skillet. Cook for 5 minutes or until the sauce thickens. Remove from heat.
4. To serve, spoon equal amounts into lettuce leaves.

Fish Tofu and Shrimps Stir-Fry

Ingredients:

- 1 package fish tofu, halved
- 1 ½ pounds shrimp, uncooked
- 1 white onion, minced
- 2 garlic cloves, minced
- ¼ pound French beans
- 1 tablespoon olive oil
- Pinch of sea salt

For the Cornstarch slurry

- tablespoon cornstarch
- ¼ cup water
- 1 tablespoon oyster sauce
- ¼ teaspoon palm sugar, crumbled

Directions:

1. Mix salt and shrimps in a bowl.
2. Mix cornstarch slurry in another bowl until sugar dissolves.
3. Pour oil into non-stick wok set over high heat; sauté garlic and onion until limp and transparent.
4. Add in fish tofu and shrimps; stir-fry until latter turns coral. Add in remaining ingredients, including cornstarch slurry; cook until sauce thickens and French beans turn a shade brighter, about 3 minutes. Turn off heat immediately. Taste; adjust seasoning if needed. Spoon equal portions into plates; serve.

All Mushrooms Bake

Ingredients:

- 2 cups mixed wild mushrooms
- 1 cup chestnut mushrooms
- 2 cups dried porcini
- 2 shallots
- 4 garlic cloves
- 3 cups raw pecans
- ½ bunch fresh thyme
- 1 bunch flat-leaf parsley
- 2 tablespoons olive oil
- 2 fresh bay leaves
- 1 ½ cups stale bread

Directions:

1. Remove skin and finely chop garlic and shallots. Roughly chop the wild mushrooms and chestnut mushrooms. Pick the leaves of the thyme and tear the bread into small pieces. Put inside the pressure cooker.
2. Place the pecans and roughly chop the nuts. Pick the parsley leaves and roughly chop.
3. Place the porcini in a bowl and add 300ml of boiling water. Set aside until needed.
4. Heat oil in the pressure cooker. Add the garlic and shallots. Cook for 3 minutes while stirring occasionally.
5. Drain porcini and reserve the liquid. Add the porcini into the pressure cooker together with the wild mushrooms and chestnut mushrooms. Add the bay leaves and thyme.
6. Position the lid and lock in place. Put to high heat and bring

to high pressure. Adjust heat to stabilize. Cook for 10 minutes. Adjust taste if necessary.
7. Transfer the mushroom mixture into a bowl and set aside to cool completely.
8. Once the mushrooms are completely cool, add the bread, pecans, a pinch of black pepper and sea salt, and half of the reserved liquid into the bowl. Mix well. Add more reserved liquid if the mixture seems dry.
9. Add more than half of the parsley into the bowl and stir. Transfer the mixture into a 20cm x 25cm lightly greased baking dish and cover with tin foil.
10. Bake in the oven for 35 minutes. Then, remove the foil and cook for another 10 minutes. Once done, sprinkle the remaining parsley on top and serve with bread or crackers. Serve.

Zucchini Roll-ups

Ingredients:
Cream cheese

- 1 tsp. sour cream
- ¼ cup cream cheese
- ⅛ cup fresh chives, minced
- Pinch of sea salt
- Pinch of white pepper

———-

- 2 zucchini, shave into long and wide slivers
- ¼ pound ham, thinly sliced

Directions:

1. In a small mixing bowl, combine cream cheese, chives, sour cream, salt, and pepper. Mix until all ingredients are well combined.
2. Put zucchini slivers on a flat surface. Spread the cream cheese mix. Sprinkle ham. Roll into tight bundles and secure with toothpicks. Serve.

Artichoke, Beef and Bell Peppers Pie

Ingredients:

For the Pie Filling

- 1 artichoke hearts, diced
- 1 green bell pepper, diced
- 1 red bell pepper, diced
- ½ cup lean ground beef
- 1 garlic clove, minced
- 1/16 tsp. cumin powder
- Pinch of sea salt
- Pinch of white pepper
- 1 Tbsp. olive oil

Directions:

1. Preheat the oven to 350 degrees F.
2. For the pie filling, heat the oil into a non-stick skillet. Saute the garlic for 3 minutes or until fragrant.

1. Stir in ground beef. Cook until the meat becomes brown and larger clumps are broken into small pieces.
2. Put green bell and red bell pepper artichoke hearts, cumin powder, salt, and pepper into the Dutch oven. Stir well. Adjust seasoning if needed.
3. For the pies, put just the right amount of pie filling into oven-safe ramekins.
4. Put ramekins on a baking sheet and bake for 20 minutes. Serve.

Chili Mushroom and Beans

Ingredients:

- ½ pound shiitake mushrooms, dried, soaked in water for 2 hours, reserve...
- 1 cup mushroom's soaking liquid
- 1 cup dried black beans, soaked in water overnight
- 2 red chili peppers, minced
- ¼ cup mustard seeds
- ½ cup cashew cheese
- ½ cup coconut cream
- 1 can diced tomatoes
- 3 cups vegetable broth
- 1½ tsp. cumin powder
- ¼ cup water
- 1 can tomato paste
- 2 Tbsp. paprika powder
- ½ tsp. cardamom powder

- ¼ cup fresh cilantro, minced
- 1 lime, wedged, pips removed

Directions:

1. Except for garnishes, coconut cream and cashew cheese, pour remaining ingredients into crock pot set at medium heat setting. Season lightly. Stir. Put lid on. Cook for 5 hours undisturbed.

2. Turn off heat. Add in cashew cheese and coconut cream. Stir. Taste. Adjust seasoning if needed.
3. Ladle chili into individual portions. Garnish with 1 slice of lime and cilantro, if using. Squeeze lime juice on top before eating.

Mushrooms Ziti Marinara

Ingredients:

- 2 cups wholegrain ziti, uncooked
- 1 cup dried shiitake mushrooms, soaked in water for 3 hours, quartered, reserve...
- 1 cup mushroom soaking liquid
- 1 cup water
- 1½ cups marinara sauce
- 3 garlic cloves, minced
- 1 onion, minced
- 1 eggplant, diced
- 2 tsp. sea salt
- 1 tsp. black pepper
- 1 tsp. olive oil
- fresh basil, minced, for garnish

Directions:

1. Pour oil into Dutch oven set over medium heat. Add in eggplant and sauté until seared well on all sides. Add in onion, garlic, and a small pinch of salt. Stir fry for another 1 minute.
2. Except for basil, add remaining ingredients into Dutch oven. Put lid partially on. Let this come to a gently boil, stirring often. Cook only until ziti is al dente. Turn off heat.
3. Ladle dish into individual portions. Sprinkle basil on top. Serve warm.

Halibut Egg Rolls

Ingredients:

Dipping sauce

- Pinch of sea salt to taste
- ½ teaspoon white pepper
- 2 tablespoons fish sauce
- ⅛ cup rice wine vinegar
- 4 tablespoons packed palm sugar, crumbled
- 2 tablespoons tomato catsup

———————-

- 8 pieces spring roll wrappers
- Olive oil
- water, for sealing

Filling

- ½ pound halibut fillets
- 8 pieces asparagus
- 1 can sliced bamboo shoots, drained
- 2 tablespoons fresh cilantro, minced
- 2 tablespoons fresh chives, minced
- ½ tablespoons light soy sauce
- Dash of white pepper

Directions:

1. Combine dipping sauce ingredients in a bowl. Stir until sugar dissolves. Taste; adjust seasoning if needed.

2. Season halibut fillets with soy sauce and white pepper. Place a fillet on 1 corner of spring roll wrapper. Add equal portions of asparagus, bamboo shoots, chives, and cilantro on top. Roll tightly, folding in edges, and sealing with water. Set aside. Repeat step for remaining ingredients.
3. Half-fill deep fryer with oil set at medium heat; wait for oil to become slightly smoky before sliding in spring rolls. Cook only until spring rolls turn golden brown, 5 to 7 minutes. Transfer cooked spring rolls to a plate lined with paper towels. Place 2 spring rolls on a plate; serve with dipping sauce on the side.

Fish Heads Stew

Ingredients:

- 4 fresh grouper fish heads
- 1 shallot, quartered
- 2 garlic cloves, crushed
- 12 okra, halved
- 2 lemongrass, knotted
- 2 string beans, sliced into inch-long pieces
- 2 celery stalks, chopped
- 2 tomatoes, chopped
- 2 Tbsp. tamarind paste
- 1 ripe pineapple, sliced into large chunks
- water, enough to submerge fish heads
- fish sauce
- black pepper, to taste
- 2 bird's eye chili, minced
- ¼ cup cilantro, torn, for garnish

Directions:

1. Layer ingredients into large stockpot, starting with: pineapples, lemongrass, string beans, okra, celery, tomatoes, garlic cloves, and shallots.
2. Place fish heads on top, preferably **not** overlapping each other.
3. Except for garnishes and tamarind paste, add in remaining ingredients. Pour just enough water to submerge fish heads.
4. Set stockpot on highest heat setting. Let this come to a boil, partially covered.
5. Turn down heat to lowest setting. Secure lid. Simmer stew for 30 to 45 minutes, or until fish skin is fork tender. Do not stir.

Turn off heat.
6. Ladle fish heads into separate bowls. Dilute tamarind paste into fish broth. Stir to combine. Adjust seasoning, if needed. (Simply pour in lime juice, is using. Add more for a tart stew.)
7. Ladle fruits, vegetables, and fish broth into bowl with fish heads. Sprinkle cilantro and chili on top, if using. Serve immediately.

White Beans and Spinach on Wholegrain Pasta

Ingredients:

- 3 cups wholegrain, uncooked
- 1 can white beans
- 5 cups baby spinach
- 4 cups water
- ½ cup mushroom stock
- 2 Tbsp. garlic infused olive oil
- kosher salt
- white pepper, to taste

Directions:

1. Pour water into Dutch oven set over high heat. Add in a pinch of kosher salt. Put lid on. Let water come to a boil.
2. Add in pasta and cook until *al dente*. Except for 1 cup, discard boiling water.
3. Add in white beans and vegetable broth into Dutch oven. Cook only until beans are heated through, about 2 minutes. Turn off heat. Stir in baby spinach leaves into pasta. Season with salt and pepper accordingly.
4. To serve, ladle dish into individual portions. Drizzle with garlic infused olive oil. Serve warm.

Mixed Vegetables and Chicken Egg Rolls

Ingredients:

Dipping sauce

- 1 tablespoon garlic, grated
- 1 tablespoon ginger, grated
- 4 tablespoons palm sugar, crumbled
- 1 banana chili, minced
- 4 tablespoons fish sauce
- Pinch of black pepper
- 4 tablespoons rice wine vinegar
- 1 bird's eye chili, minced

―――-

- 8 pieces spring roll wrappers
- Olive oil
- water, for sealing

Filling

- 1 garlic clove, minced
- 1 shallot, julienned
- ¼ cup chicken, cooked, shredded
- 1 cup bean sprouts
- 1 tablespoon chicken concentrate
- 2 tablespoon coconut oil
- ¼ cup squash, julienned
- ¼ cup carrots, julienned
- ¼ cup sweet potato, julienned
- ¼ cup potato, julienned

- ½ cup water
- Pinch of sea salt
- Pinch of black pepper

Directions:

1. Combine dipping sauce ingredients in a bowl. Stir until sugar dissolves. Taste; adjust seasoning if needed. Set aside.
2. To make spring rolls: pour coconut oil into large wok set over medium heat. Sauté garlic and shallot until limp and transparent; except for bean sprouts, add in remaining filling ingredients. Cook until root crops are fork tender. Toss in bean sprouts; stir. Turn off heat immediately. Allow filling to cool completely to room temperature before rolling.
3. Add equal portions of vegetable filling into spring roll paper; roll tightly, tucking in the edges and sealing with water. Set aside. Repeat step for remaining filling/wrapper.
4. Half-fill deep fryer with cooking oil set at medium heat; wait for oil to become slightly smoky before sliding in spring rolls. Cook only until spring rolls turn golden brown, about 7 minutes. Transfer cooked pieces on plate lined with paper towels. Place 2 spring rolls on a plate; serve with dipping sauce on the side.

Squash and Lentils Soup

Ingredients:

- 1 butternut squash, chopped
- 1 white onion, minced
- 1 cup dried yellow lentils
- 2 carrots, grated
- 4 leeks, roots removed, minced
- 4 cups water
- 2 cups vegetable stock
- Pinch of kosher salt
- Pinch of black pepper, to taste
- 1 tsp. olive oil
- ⅛ cup fresh parsley, minced
- ¼ cup cashew cream

Directions:

1. Pour oil into large stockpot set over high heat. Add in carrots, leeks, and onions. Sauté until vegetables are limp and lightly golden.
2. Except for garnishes, add in remaining ingredients into pot. Let liquids come to a boil. Put lid on.
3. Turn down heat to lowest setting. Let soup simmer for 30 to 35 minutes, or until squash and lentils are almost mushy. Season lightly with salt and pepper.
4. You can serve soup as is, or if you want a smoother texture, process soup using an immersion blender.
5. Ladle into individual portions. Place a small amount of cashew cream on top, then a pinch of minced parsley, if using. Serve warm.

Halibut Tortilla Tacos with Tartar Sauce

Ingredients:
For the Fish

- 1½ pounds halibut fillets, sliced into slivers
- 1 cup breadcrumbs
- ½ tsp. sweet paprika powder
- 2 eggs, whisked
- ½ cup all-purpose flour
- ¼ tsp. cayenne pepper
- Pinch of salt
- Pinch of black pepper

- 8 pieces wheat tortilla bread, warmed
- 2 lime, sliced into equal wedges

For the Tartar Sauce

- 1 cup mayonnaise, reduced fat
- ½ cup cilantro, minced
- 2 Tbsp. capers in brine
- ¼ cup parsley, minced
- 2 Tbsp. lemon juice, freshly squeezed

- Avocado slices
- 1 tomato, sliced
- Cabbage, shredded

Directions:

1. Season halibut fillet slivers with salt, black pepper, sweet paprika, and cayenne pepper. Set aside to drain in a colander for 15 minutes.
2. Meanwhile, in a bowl, combined flour, eggs, and panko breadcrumbs into three separate bowls.
3. Dredge halibut fillet into this order: flour first, egg, and then coat with breadcrumbs. Place on a baking sheet. Repeat the same procedure for the remaining fillets.
4. Heat the olive oil in a non-stick skillet. Once the oil is hot and smoky, slide breaded fillets. Deep fry until golden brown. Drain on paper towels.
5. For the tartar sauce, put together capers in brine, mayonnaise, parsley, cilantro, and lemon juice in a bowl.
6. To serve, place fish fillets into soft tacos. Add in cabbage, avocadoes, and tomatoes. Put a dollop of tartar sauce. Squeeze lime juice over. Serve.

Turkey Breast in Tomato Sauce

Ingredients:

- 1 cup turkey breast, boneless, skinless, cubed
- ¾ cup tomato sauce
- ½ teaspoon hot pepper sauce
- 1 teaspoon extra virgin olive oil
- ½ teaspoon ground cloves
- ½ cup onion, chopped finely
- ¼ teaspoon mustard powder
- Pinch of pepper
- 2 cups spinach, cooked

Directions:

1. Heat olive oil in a saucepan set over medium heat. Saute onion for 3 minutes or until the onion starts to soften.
2. Add in mustard, tomato sauce, hot pepper sauce, ground cloves, and pepper. Reduce heat and allow to simmer for 5 minutes.
3. To serve, divide cooked spinach in plates. Pour cooked marinated turkey breast.

Chapter 9 – Desserts/ Snacks

Blueberry Scones

Ingredients:

- 1 cup blueberries
- 1 cup ground whole oats
- 1 ¼ cups whole grain pastry flour
- 2 tablespoons ground flaxseeds
- ½ teaspoon baking soda
- 2 teaspoons baking powder
- 1 cup plain yogurt
- ½ cup dairy milk, nonfat
- Pinch of salt
- 2 tablespoons lemon juice
- 2 tablespoons olive oil

Directions:

1. Preheat the oven to 400 degrees F. Lightly grease a baking sheet.
2. In a bowl, put together baking soda, baking powder oats flaxseed, salt, and milk.
3. In a separate bowl, whisk together yogurt, olive oil, lemon zest, and lemon juice.
4. Make a well in the center of the dry ingredients and pour the yogurt mixture. Stir in blueberries. Stir well.
5. Drop batter onto the baking sheet. Bake for 15 minutes. Serve

Vegan Ice Cream, Vanilla Flavor

Ingredients:

- cup light coconut milk
- 3/4 tsp vanilla bean paste
- 1/3 cup agave nectar
- 2/3 cup soy milk

Directions:

1. Combine all of the ingredients in a mixing bowl, then pour it into an ice cream maker.
2. Set the ice cream maker to churn for 30 minutes, then transfer the mixture into a container and place it in the freezer
3. Let the ice cream freeze for a minimum of 4 hours, then serve.

Banana Choco Cookies

Ingredients:

- 3 ripe bananas, pureed
- 1 cup dark chocolate chips
- 2 eggs, whisked
- ½ cup coconut flour, finely milled
- 3 cups almond flour, coarsely milled
- 1 tsp. vanilla extract
- 1 tsp. cinnamon powder
- ¼ cup coconut flakes, unsweetened

Directions:

1. Preheat the oven to 350°F (175°C). Line a baking sheet with parchment paper.
2. Meanwhile, in a large mixing bowl, put together bananas, almond flour, coconut flour, cinnamon powder, coconut flakes, vanilla extract, and applesauce. Pour contents into the Instant Pot Pressure Cooker.
3. Press "steam" button. Mix mixture well. Fold in chocolate chips. Allow mixture to come together for 4 minutes, whilst stirring frequently.
4. Turn off the heat and let cool for 3 minutes. Put a generous amount of batter on the baking sheet. Bake for 25 minutes or until the edges are set and golden in color.
5. Place cookies on the cake rack and let cool before serving.

Pecan Cilantro Pancakes

Ingredients:

- 4 cups pecan flour, finely milled
- ½ cup cilantro leaves, minced
- 2 ½ cups water
- Pinch of kosher salt
- ½ cup coconut oil
- salsa, store-bought, for dipping

Directions:

1. Combine dipping sauce in small bowl. Set aside
2. Lightly grease a large non-stick skillet with coconut oil; set aside.
3. Mix remaining ingredients in a bowl until dough comes together. Turn out dough on lightly floured flat surface; knead until elastic.
4. Divide into 8 equal portions; roll into balls, tucking in edges underneath to make dough look seamless. Using a rolling pin, flatten each out to roughly the size of skillet's cooking surface.
5. Set skillet over medium heat. Fry flat breads one at a time until small pockets of air develops within; flip and continue cooking until lightly brown on both sides. Place cooked pieces on a serving platter lined with tea towel.
6. Using pastry brush, lightly grease both sides of flat bread with oil. Cover platter with another tea towel to prevent bread from drying out. Repeat step until all flat breads are cooked.
7. Place 2 pieces on plates; slice these into wedges. Serve with desired amount of dipping sauce on the side.

Cashew Cheese

Ingredients:

- 1 cup raw cashew nuts, soaked in water for 1 hour, rinsed, drained
- 2 garlic cloves, minced
- 1 Tbsp. Dijon mustard
- 2 Tbsp. lemon juice, freshly squeezed
- 2 Tbsp. apple cider vinegar
- Pinch of salt
- Pinch of white pepper, to taste
- ¼ cup water

Directions:

1. Place ingredients into the pressure cooker.
2. Position the lid and lock in place.
3. Put to high heat and bring to high pressure. Adjust heat to stabilize. Cook for 5 minutes. Let cool.
4. Transfer to the food processor. Process until smooth. Season lightly. Spread on toast.

Sausage and Beans Tacos

Ingredients:

- 4 corn tortilla shells
- ½ lb sausage, crumbled
- 3 tablespoons canned black beans
- 3 tablespoons canned corn kernels
- 3 tablespoons cheddar cheese, shredded
- 2/3 cup lettuce, shredded
- 3 tablespoons salsa
- 1 teaspoon lemon juice, freshly squeezed
- ¼ teaspoon chili powder
- Olive oil

Directions:

1. Put together black beans, corn kernels, salsa, and cheddar cheese in a bowl. Mix well until all ingredients are well-combined.
2. Meanwhile, heat the olive oil in a skillet. Cook vegetarian sausage for 2 minutes. Squeeze in lemon juice and a bit of chili powder.
3. Divide cooked sausage mixture among tortilla shells. Put the bean-corn salsa. Top with shredded lettuce. Serve.

Rosemary Flat Bread

Ingredients:

- ½ cup rosemary, minced
- 3 cups coconut flour, finely milled
- 2 ½ cups water
- 1 cup all-purpose flour
- ½ cup coconut oil, melted
- Pinch of kosher salt

Dipping sauce

- ¼ teaspoons pomegranate vinegar
- ¼ pound ripe tomatoes, minced
- Pinch of salt
- Pinch of white pepper

Directions:

1. Combine dipping sauce in small bowl. Set aside
2. Lightly grease a large non-stick skillet with coconut oil; set aside.
3. Mix remaining ingredients in a bowl until dough comes together. Turn out dough on lightly floured flat surface; knead until elastic. Divide into 8 equal portions; roll into balls, tucking in edges underneath to make dough look seamless. Using a rolling pin, flatten each out to roughly the size of skillet's cooking surface.
4. Set skillet over medium heat. Fry flat breads one at a time until small pockets of air develops within; flip and continue cooking until lightly brown on both sides. Place cooked pieces

on a serving platter lined with tea towel.
5. Using pastry brush, lightly grease both sides of flat bread with oil. Cover platter with another tea towel to prevent bread from drying out. Repeat step until all flat breads are cooked.
6. Place 2 pieces on plates; slice these into wedges. Serve with desired amount of dipping sauce on the side.

Minty Cranberry Iced Tea

Ingredients:

- 3½ cups water
- 8 tea bags black tea

- 2 cups water
- ¾ cup palm sugar, crumbled
- ¼ cup mint leaves
- 2 pears, diced
- ½ pound cranberries
- icy water

Directions:

1. To prepare tea: pour water into saucepan set over high heat. Boil. Turn off heat. Add in tea bags. Secure lid; and steep tea for 10 minutes. Discard tea bags.
2. To prepare infusion: pour water and sugar into the other saucepan set over medium heat. Cook until sugar dissolves. Turn off heat. Mix in mint, and steep in syrup for 10 minutes. Place fruits in a Mason jar. Strain syrup into fruits.
3. Discard spent mint. Pour in prepared tea. Fill a Mason jar with icy water until almost full. Mix. Secure lid. Chill drink for at least an hour before serving.
4. To serve: pour iced tea into tall glasses. Serve.

Squash and Tomato Pate

Ingredients:

- 1 can butternut squash puree
- ¼ cup sun-dried tomatoes
- ⅛ tsp. garlic powder
- ⅛ tsp. onion powder
- ½ cup vegetable stock, warmed
- ⅛ tsp. Spanish paprika
- Pinch of salt
- Pinch of white pepper, to taste
- 1 Tbsp. extra virgin olive oil

Directions:

1. Pour ingredients into the pressure cooker.
2. Position the lid and lock in place. Put to high heat and bring to high pressure. Adjust heat to stabilize. Cook for 5 minutes. Let cool.
3. Transfer to the food processor. Process until smooth. Season lightly. Spread on toast.

Grapefruit and Apricot Iced Tea

Ingredients:

For the tea

- 8 tea bags black tea
- 3½ cups water

For infusion

- 2 apricots, cubed
- 1 grapefruit, pulp only
- ⅛ cup cardamom pods, lightly crushed
- 2 cups water
- ¾ cup palm sugar, crumbled
- icy water

Directions:

1. To prepare tea: pour water into saucepan set over high heat. Boil. Turn off heat. Add in tea bags. Secure lid; and steep tea for 10 minutes. Discard tea bags.
2. To prepare infusion: pour water and sugar into the other saucepan set over medium heat. Cook until sugar dissolves. Turn off heat. Mix in cardamom pods, and steep in syrup for 10 minutes. Place fruits in a Mason jar. Strain syrup into fruits.
3. Discard cardamom pods. Pour in prepared tea. Fill a Mason jar with icy water until almost full. Mix. Secure lid. Chill drink for at least an hour before serving.
4. To serve: pour iced tea into tall glasses. Serve.

Blueberry-Banana Hotcakes

Ingredients:

- ½ cup blueberries
- 1 ripe banana, mashed
- 2 eggs, yolks and whites separated
- 1 cup coconut flour, finely milled
- 2 unsweetened applesauce
- ¼ cup water
- ¼ tsp. coconut oil

Directions:

1. Beat the egg whites. Set aside.
2. Using another medium-sized mixing bowl, put together egg yolks, applesauce, water, coconut flour, banana, and half of the blueberries. Mix well until a thick consistency is achieved. Fold in the egg whites.
3. Using the Instant Pot Pressure Cooker. Press the "saute" button and heat the coconut oil. Once the oil is hot, drop an equal amount of batter. Cook for 1 minute or until a bubble forms on top. Flip to the other side and cook for 1 more minute.
4. Cook in batches until all hotcakes are cooked. Garnish with the remaining blueberries. Serve.

Cranberry and Mango Iced Tea

Ingredients:

- 3½ cups water
- 8 tea bags black tea

For the infusion

- ½ pound cranberries
- 1 ripe mango, cubed
- ¼ cup mint leaves
- 2 cups water
- ¾ cup palm sugar, crumbled
- icy water

Directions:

1. To prepare tea: pour water into saucepan set over high heat. Boil. Turn off heat. Add in tea bags. Secure lid; and steep tea for 10 minutes. Discard tea bags.
2. To prepare infusion: pour water and sugar into the other saucepan set over medium heat. Cook until sugar dissolves. Turn off heat. Mix in mint, and steep in syrup for 10 minutes. Place fruits in a Mason jar. Strain syrup into fruits.

Minty Strawberry Iced Tea

Ingredients:

- 4 cups water
- 8 tea bags black tea

For the infusion

- 1 pound strawberries
- 1 cup mint leaves
- ¾ cup palm sugar, crumbled
- 1 cup water
- icy water

Directions:

1. To prepare tea: pour water into saucepan set over high heat. Boil. Turn off heat. Add in tea bags. Secure lid; and steep tea for 10 minutes. Discard tea bags.
2. To prepare infusion: pour water and sugar into the other saucepan set over medium heat. Cook until sugar dissolves. Turn off heat. Mix in mint, and steep in syrup for 10 minutes.
3. Place fruits in a Mason jar. Strain syrup into fruits. Discard spent mint. Pour in prepared tea. Fill a Mason jar with icy water until almost full. Mix. Secure lid. Chill drink for at least an hour before serving.
4. To serve: pour iced tea into tall glasses. Serve.

Mash Potato and Carrot

Ingredients:

- 2 potatoes, cubed
- 3 carrots, cubed
- ½ cup half-and-half
- 1¼ cups Parmigiano-Reggiano, grated
- 1/16 tsp. cumin powder
- 1 Tbsp. lemon juice, freshly squeezed
- 2 cups water
- 2 Tbsp. salt
- 1/16 tsp. black pepper

Directions:

1. Pour water into a Dutch oven. Place potatoes and carrots. Season with salt. Bring to a boil.
2. Reduce the heat and allow to simmer for 20 minutes or until the vegetables are tender.
3. Turn off the heat. Drain water.
4. Pour half and half, Parmigiano-Reggiano, cumin powder, lemon juice, and black pepper into the Dutch oven.
5. Place cooked potatoes and carrots into the potato masher and process vegetables until creamy. Adjust seasoning if needed. Serve.

Basil Strawberry Iced Tea

Ingredients:

- 4½ cups water
- 8 tea bags black tea

For infusion

- 1 cup fresh basil leaves
- 1 pound strawberries
- 1 cup water
- ¾ cup palm sugar, crumbled
- icy water

Directions:

1. To prepare tea: pour water into saucepan set over high heat. Boil. Turn off heat. Add in tea bags. Secure lid; and steep tea for 10 minutes. Discard tea bags.
2. To prepare infusion: pour water and sugar into the other saucepan set over medium heat. Cook until sugar dissolves. Turn off heat. Mix in basil, and steep in syrup for 10 minutes. Place fruits in a Mason jar. Strain syrup into fruits.
3. Discard spent basil. Pour in prepared tea. Fill a Mason jar with icy water until almost full. Mix. Secure lid. Chill drink for at least an hour before serving.
4. To serve: pour iced tea into tall glasses. Serve.

Dark Coco and Walnuts Bites

Ingredients:

- 2 1/2 tbsp. dark chocolate chips
- 2 1/2 tbsp. cocoa powder
- 2 1/2 tbsp. walnuts, chopped
- 1/2 cup dates, chopped finely
- 2 1/2 tbsp. sesame seeds
- 1/4 tsp vanilla extract
- 1/4 tsp cinnamon
- 1/8 tsp sea salt

Directions:

1. Simply combine all of the ingredients in a food processor or blender and pulse until it becomes a thick paste.
2. With a tablespoon, scoop out the paste and form into balls. Arrange the balls on a tray that could fit inside your freezer.
3. Once the entire mixture has been divided into balls, freeze them for at least 20 minutes. Serve chilled and store any excess in a covered container in the freezer for up to 2 weeks.

Breadless Pizza

Ingredients:

Pizza

- 1 pound ground beef
- 1 garlic clove, grated
- 2 eggs, whisked
- 1 can diced tomatoes
- 1 tsp. oregano powder
- 3 Tbsp. raw almond slivers
- 3 Tbsp. Parmesan cheese, grated
- 3 Tbsp. fresh parsley, minced
- 1 cup fresh basil leaves, torn
- 4 oz mozzarella balls, sliced thinly
- Pinch of sea salt
- Pinch of black pepper

Directions:

1. Preheat the oven to 425 degrees °F. Lightly grease a baking tin with cooking spray. Set aside.
2. Meanwhile, in a large mixing bowl, put together ground beef, garlic clove, eggs, oregano powder, almond slivers, Parmesan cheese, and parsley. Season with salt and pepper. Mix well. Press the mixture onto the baking sheet.
3. Spread tomatoes on top of the mixture. Sprinkle basil and put mozzarella balls.
4. Bake for 30 minutes or until lightly browned. Remove from the tin and allow to sit for 5 minutes before slicing.

Chapter 10 - Frequently Asked Questions

Q: Won't I get really hungry if I decide to fast for 24 hours?

A: You won't. You can actually live without food for 30 days. You just have to keep yourself hydrated. Based on studies, a well-hydrated person who doesn't eat anything won't die of starvation even if the fasting stretches for 30 days. Death without food only occurs within the 45th - 60th day. So, yes, you're still okay for 1-30 days. Of course, before you decide on fasting for as long as 30 days, you have to consult your doctor about it and make sure you don't have a serious medical condition.

Q: Is Intermittent Fasting dangerous?

A: No. If you're a healthy person. Fasting for 16 or more hours won't lead to starvation, but expect that you'll feel weak and grumpy the whole time. According to medical experts, fasting is safe for the body and offers good benefits. Again, do not fast if you're not physically well.

Q: Is it okay to eat small frequent meals for the whole day?

A: Yes, you may eat small amount of food every three hours. This is to rev up your metabolism and burn more calories. In order to burn fats, you'll have to use up all glucose in the body first, and this is only made possible by fasting.

Q: Can I still fast even if I workout?

A: Yes, you can. First, you have to find the most convenient fasting period for you. Do light exercises first and then gradually introduce the body to more challenging workouts. Don't forget to keep yourself hydrated at all times.

If you feel weak, you may skip your workout and just focus on fasting until your body gets used to the routine of fasting and working out all at the same time. Check the food you eat as well and make sure to have enough protein in your everyday diet.

Conclusion

Thank you again for downloading this book.

This book contains basic guidelines on how to safely start Intermittent Fasting. Aside from the steps on what you should do, there are also recommendations on how to start your own Intermittent Fasting schedule and recipes that you can try, and so much more.

The next step is to make your own Intermittent Fasting schedule so that you can lose weight effectively and successfully.

Thank you and good luck!

Other Books By Susanne Bernard

Did you enjoy this book?

I want to thank you for purchasing and reading this book. I really hope you got a lot out of it.

Thanks so much.

Susanne Bernard

ALL RIGHTS RESERVED. No part of this publication may be reproduced or transmitted in any form whatsoever, electronic, or mechanical, including photocopying, recording, or by any informational storage or retrieval system without express written, dated and signed permission from the author.